MW00583618

HEALTHY LIVING SERIES: 3 BOOKS IN 1

7 STEPS TO GET OFF SUGAR AND CARBOHYDRATES;
CHRISTIAN STUDY GUIDE FOR 7 STEPS TO GET OFF
SUGAR AND CARBOHYDRATES; HEALTHY LIVING
JOURNAL

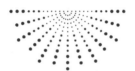

SUSAN U. NEAL RN, MBA, MHS

CHRISTIAN INDIE
PUBLISHING

Editor: Janis Whipple

Cover Design: Angie Alaya

ISBN: 978-1-733-64430-3

Printed in the United States of America

INTRODUCTION

I am excited you decided to take this journey of health and wellness. Nine years ago I lost my health with ten medical diagnoses and two surgeries. I had to fight to regain it. Now I am on a mission to help others reclaim their health and weight so they can live the abundant life God planned for them.

To support you along this journey, I created a closed Facebook group, 7 Steps to Get Off Sugar, Carbs, and Gluten. Please join this group and let me know how you are doing. In this group, I am available to answer your questions.

Many individuals have found health and healing by applying the principles in this book. We should eat God's natural foods, not the food manufacturers. Evaluate everything you eat and make sure it came from the garden or farm.

Processed foods packaged in boxes and bags are convenient. Unfortunately, the nutrients our Creator put into fruits, vegetables, and grains get stripped away as these packaged foods are processed, so they can be stored on the grocery shelves for months, if not years.

Therefore, we starve ourselves of essential nutrients the body requires to be healthy. No wonder over half of Americans live with a chronic illness. Apparently, we are not eating the foods God designed, but the foods manufacturers create for their profit.

If you overeat, crave the wrong type of foods, or eat in a manner you do not like *Healthy Living Series: 3 Books in 1* will help you figure out the root source of an inappropriate eating habit. The top four reasons include:

- Lack of knowledge
- Candida overgrowth
- Food addiction
- Emotional connection with food

One reason it is difficult for many to stick to decisions about food is that their bodies betray their mental commitment. That's why this book will explain how addictions affect us physically, so we can be prepared with the mental ammunition needed to stay strong. Sweets and refined carbohydrates are addictive and harmful to the human body. That is why 40 percent of Americans suffer from obesity. This book provides step-by-step instructions on how to stop the cravings and unwanted symptoms associated with eating a diet loaded with carbs.

We will also explore the possibility of a candida infection of the gut. You will gain an understanding of the types of food to avoid and why. Once you have the knowledge you need to make the right decision for your health, you'll be better equipped to make the next step, and the next, until you've changed your lifestyle. With your lifestyle change, you will live the abundant life Jesus wants you to experience, not a life filled with disease and unwanted, unhealthy symptoms.

This book will help you understand what may be causing your issues and how to resolve it. Deciding is the first step to transformation. Begin by asking God to make you willing to change. Once you are willing, write down the changes you will make, and commit to them before the Lord. Ask God to help you and place your success in his loving arms.

Healthy Living Series: 3 Books in 1 includes the following three books in the Healthy Living Series:

- *7 Steps to Get Off Sugar and Carbohydrates*
- *Christian Study Guide for 7 Steps to Get Off Sugar and Carbohydrates*
- *Healthy Living Journal*

Initially I wrote *7 Steps to Get Off Sugar and Carbohydrates,* but I found that my readers needed to go deeper. So I published *Christian Study Guide for 7 Steps to Get Off Sugar and Carbohydrates* to reinforce the principles from the first book.

Through the Christian study guide, you will learn how to utilize God's divine power to evoke lifelong changes rather than rely on self-control. This book differs from other healthy living books because we learn to equip ourselves with spiritual weapons to attain victory.

This plan is not a diet but a lifestyle change. However, the guidelines are not so stringent that you feel like you have a noose around your neck. You apply God's wisdom along with accurate knowledge about today's food.

The third book in the series, *Healthy Living Journal* helps you record daily water intake, exercise, and corresponding moods and energy. Recording your daily food consumption provides an opportunity to learn how food affects your health. This will help you figure out what type of food makes your body function well or poorly. When you discover negative health patterns you can change.

Devotions and educational snippets are provided daily in the journal. Learn about food addiction, Candida infection of the gut, and healthy eating guidelines from these daily entries. As you gain knowledge, you will learn how to improve your health and weight. You will also journal and spend time with God. You are a child of God and deserve the most life has to offer you. Choose to take the time needed to improve your health; your body will thank you.

I also created the Healthy Living Blog to provide you with helpful articles, menus, recipes, and lifestyle tips. You can subscribe to it at SusanUNeal.com/Healthy-Living-Blog.

In addition, feel free to join my closed Facebook group: 7 Steps to Get Off Sugar, Carbs, and Gluten and let me know how you are doing. In this group, I am available to answer all of your questions. I have another Facebook page, Healthy Living Series, to keep you up to date with relevant information about maintaining a healthy lifestyle at Facebook.com/HealthyLivingSeries/.

If you need additional support making this lifestyle change, purchase my course, 7 Steps to Reclaim Your Health and Optimal Weight. In this course I walk you through all the material covered in my Healthy Living Series. I help you change your eating habits once and for all.

You are about to embark on a journey to improve the stewardship of your body. You only have one body, and it needs to last a lifetime. May God bless your endeavor to improve your health.

7 STEPS TO GET OFF SUGAR AND CARBOHYDRATES

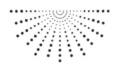

HEALTHY EATING FOR HEALTHY LIVING WITH A LOW-CARBOHYDRATE, ANTI-INFLAMMATORY DIET

I would like to dedicate this book to my sister, Kim. I am proud of you for getting off sugar and refined carbohydrates. Thank you for allowing me to share your story so that others may benefit from it. May God bless you.

DISCLAIMER

Medical Disclaimer: This book offers health and nutritional information, which is for educational purposes only. The information provided in this book is designed to help individuals make informed decisions about their health; it is intended to supplement, not replace, the professional medical advice, diagnosis, or treatment of health conditions from a trained medical professional. Please consult your physician or healthcare provider before beginning or changing any health or eating habits to make sure that it is appropriate for you. If you have any concerns or questions about your health, you should always ask a physician or other healthcare provider. Please do not disregard, avoid, or delay obtaining medical or health-related advice from your healthcare professional because of something you may have read in this book. The author and publisher assumes no responsibility for any injury that may result from changing your health or eating habits.

Disclaimer and Terms of Use: Every effort has been made to ensure the information in this book is accurate and complete. However, the author and publisher do not warrant the accuracy or completeness of the material, text, and graphics contained in this book. The author and publisher do not hold any responsibility for

A FREE GIFT FOR YOU

I am excited you decided to take this journey of health and wellness. To help you succeed, I included ten appendices chock-full of plans, strategies, and summarized information. To receive a printable version of the appendices please go to SusanUNeal.com/appendix.

I created the Healthy Living Blog to provide you with helpful articles, menus, recipes, and lifestyle tips. You can subscribe to it at Susan-UNeal.com/Healthy-Living-Blog.

In addition, feel free to join my closed Facebook group: 7 Steps to Get Off Sugar, Carbs, and Gluten and let me know how you are doing. In this group, I am available to answer all of your questions. I have another Facebook page, Healthy Living Series, to keep you up to date with relevant information about maintaining a healthy lifestyle at Facebook.com/HealthyLivingSeries/.

The two additional books contained in the Healthy Living Series include *Christian Study for 7 Steps to Get Off Sugar and Carbohydrates* and *Healthy Living Journal.* The mega book, *Healthy Living Series: 3 Books in 1* includes all three of the books.

If you need additional support making this lifestyle change, purchase my course, 7 Steps to Reclaim Your Health and Optimal Weight (https://susanuneal.com/courses/7-steps-to-get-off-sugar-and-carbs-course). In this course I walk you through all the material covered in my Healthy Living Series. I help you change your eating habits once and for all.

INTRODUCTION

Chronic diseases are an epidemic today, and many of them can be prevented or reversed. Excess weight and health issues may be keeping you from having a life of abundance now and in the future. Weight problems lead to other issues—lack of energy, trouble buying clothes, stress from diets, difficulty moving or keeping up with family members, physical ailments and pain, financial burdens from health-care visits and medications. Not to mention the emotional and spiritual struggles, such as self-consciousness about your appearance and how this affects the activities you choose to be involved in, or feeling you missed out on years of being who God created you to be.

If you relate to any of these struggles, would you like to improve the way you feel and look while increasing your energy level and clarity of mind? How about losing weight naturally without going on a fad diet or buying prepared meals and supplements? You can achieve these results through simply changing the types of food you eat.

As a registered nurse (RN) with a master of health science, I research and study healthy eating lifestyles to determine which foods are best for the human body. Knowing what foods to eat and avoid is essential to prevent food-related illnesses. I also understand the addictive nature of sugar and wheat and what it does to our bodies. When we consume sugar or wheat, dopamine releases in the brain, which drives us to eat more. Therefore, these products are biochemically addictive, and we must understand this so we can make the changes necessary for our health.

If anyone was addicted to sugar, it was my sister. She loved sweets. Doughnuts in the morning, soft drinks throughout the day, bread, pasta, chocolate, and candy—you get the picture. She has been overweight since she was a child. She suffered from joint pain and irritable bowel syndrome. She never knew when a specific food might set her off and she would need to be close to a bathroom for a whole day.

Being physically ill is only one aspect of how food addictions affect people. Not fitting into clothes and feeling unattractive can undermine a person's self-esteem. Then their pocketbooks are gouged, as they need to buy new clothes because the old ones don't fit. Does this sound familiar? Do you crave carbs too? When my sister was forty-nine, she asked me to help her get off sugar and carbohydrates. From my experience, this is difficult to do, so I created a seven-step plan for her to follow:

7 Steps to Get Off Sugar and Carbohydrates

1. **Decide** to improve your health through proper nutrition.
2. **Acquire** a support system and knowledge to help make a lifestyle change.
3. **Clean out** the pantry and refrigerator by removing unhealthy foods and clean out your emotions.
4. **Purchase** healthy foods plus an anti-Candida cleanse.
5. **Plan** for the start date to begin changing your eating habits.
6. **Prepare** and eat foods differently than you did before.
7. **Improve** your health through continuing this new lifestyle, never turning back to your old eating habits.

My sister not only took the seven-step plan to heart but she allowed me to share her story with you, in the hopes it will encourage you to try the plan yourself. The first time my sister tried this plan she was successful with getting off wheat because she'd tested positive for gluten sensitivity, and when she eliminated wheat her irritable bowel symptoms disappeared. This lifestyle change was easier for her because a physical pain disappeared. However, she continued to eat sugary foods, not recognizing their affect on her health. Finally, one year later, she had another health crisis, and successfully implemented the full plan.

One week after getting off sugars and refined carbohydrates, my sister's energy and rosacea skin condition improved. By the second week, her joints no longer ached, and the craving for sugar subsided. Two months later, she'd lost ten pounds and felt energized. After that, she lost five pounds per month until she got to her ideal weight and her rosacea disappeared.

If you choose to embark on this seven-step plan, you will radically improve your health and energy by merely removing sugars and refined carbohydrates. However, this plan is not a diet, where once you complete the seven steps, you're done. This is a *lifestyle change*. Typically, diets are unsuccessful because after people lose their desired weight, they go back to old eating habits, which caused them to gain weight in the first place, and find themselves facing the same challenges again and again.

The seven steps provided here are designed to incorporate your entire self—mind, body, and spirit—in making this lifestyle change so you can experience a new future, instead of another yo-yo diet that sends you back to square one. The specific instructions regarding these seven steps are provided in the next seven chapters. Each chapter begins with the following diagram, with the phase reviewed in that chapter in bold.

Decide—>Acquire—>Clean Out—>Purchase—>Plan—>Prepare—>Improve

I am excited you chose to join me on this path to wellness. God gave you a glorious body that is programmed to heal itself, if we provide it with the proper nutrition he intended. I applaud you for having the courage to take on the challenge to reclaim your body and life. I pray that God will help you and walk beside you during this journey to health.

If you have an emotional connection with food, please consider using the *Christian Study Guide for 7 Steps to Get Off Sugar and Carbohydrates.* Whether you do this study by yourself or with a group, it will help you go more in-depth to resolve an emotional issue once and for all. Please join my closed Facebook group: 7 Steps to Get Off Sugar and Carbohydrates and share with me how you are doing.

1

STEP 1: DECIDE TO IMPROVE YOUR HEALTH

Decide—>Acquire—>Clean Out—>Purchase—>Plan—>Prepare—
>Improve

If you are motivated to start making progress toward health and even weight loss, you can't skip this first step. While you may want to get right to a food list or recipes, you can't create a new lifestyle of eating and nutrition without deciding to do what is necessary to make that change. To decide is to make a definitive choice. Make a decision to commit to implementing all seven steps. Your health is worth it.

One reason it is difficult for many to stick to decisions about food is that their bodies betray their mental commitment. That's why this book will explain how addictions affect us physically, so we can be prepared with the mental ammunition needed to stay strong. Sweets and refined carbohydrates are addictive and harmful to the human body. This book provides step-by-step instructions on how to stop the cravings and unwanted symptoms associated with eating a diet loaded with carbs. We will explore the possibility of a food addiction and candida infection of the gut. You will gain an understanding of the types of food to avoid and why. Once you have the knowledge you need to make the right decision for your health, you'll be better equipped to make the next step, and the next, until you've changed your lifestyle. With your lifestyle change, you will live the abundant life Jesus wants you to experience, not a life filled with disease and unwanted, unhealthy symptoms.

THE TROUBLE WITH SUGAR AND CARBS

One of the worst carbohydrate culprits is wheat because a polypeptide in wheat crosses the blood-brain barrier, which separates the bloodstream from the brain, and binds to the brain's morphine receptors.[1] Opiate drugs (morphine, codeine, heroin, cocaine) bind to these same receptors. Unbeknownst to us, when we eat a bagel for breakfast, we consume our crack for the day.

Take the time now to watch this five-minute Ted-Ed video, "How Does Sugar Affect the Brain?" by the neuroscientist Nicole Avena, Ph.D. Go to https://www.sciencealert.com/watch-this-is-how-sugar-affects-your-brain.[2] This video explains how we get hooked on foods with a high sugar content.

As you learned from the video, sugar causes the release of dopamine in the brain, which is part of our bodies' feel-good reward system. We enjoy the feeling of dopamine, so we keep eating carbs. Sugary foods include a food item with greater than ten grams of sugar per serving. Refined carbohydrates include rice, wheat, instant mashed potatoes, instant oatmeal, cereals, potato chips, crackers, etc. At some point, an overconsumption of sugar and refined carbohydrates rewires the brain's neural pathways and causes a person to become addicted. The brain's hijacking triggers binge eating despite its consequences of weight gain and health problems. Therefore, getting off sugar is more complex than it may seem. It is no longer about willpower and self-discipline but a *biochemical addiction*. However, we can untangle the brain's rewiring to reset it back to normal, but we need to implement all the steps outlined in this book.

We live in a culture of entitlement—where we feel we deserve to satisfy ourselves to our heart's content. Countless varieties of delicious, unhealthy foods are available to us at a whim. Even the commercials on TV entice us to indulge. It is amazing that everyone in our culture has not fallen into the *food addiction trap*. Entitlement leads to indulging, which leads to addiction. It is a slippery slope once you take your first bite of that addictive food. Down the slope you fall as you consume the whole package—which you did not intend to do. If you are addicted, you can't rely on moderation. You need to understand what is causing you to consume foods in a manner you do not want to. The average American ingests up to a staggering 150 pounds of sugar each year.[3] We eat foodlike substances full of sugar and wheat, packaged in colorful, enticing boxes and bags. These so-called foods are frequently inexpensive, as well as quick and easy to prepare. We fill that immediate craving without thinking of its long-term consequences.

However, the actual cost of a steady diet of super-processed, prepackaged foods will eventually show up in chronically poor health, increased medical costs, and use of pharmaceuticals. Doctors treat the symptoms of these chronic diseases with drugs, but they usually do not address the underlying cause. Nutritious foods prevent and even reverse conditions better than expensive medications.

Over 100 million Americans suffer from chronic, painful, expensive, and often debilitating diseases. One of the dominant causes of chronic diseases in the United States is the poor quality of food consumed. When we eat processed foodstuff, we do not provide our bodies with the nutrient-filled foods God created for humans to eat.

Food industries entice consumers to eat more of their products not to improve people's health but to improve the corporations' pocketbooks. These industries put sugar in products to lure us to buy more because they understand its addictive quality. During our seven steps, you will learn about the types of food to avoid to improve your health. You'll be educated to fight back against the food industries' tactics.

NOURISH YOUR AMAZING BODY

I am intrigued with improving the functioning of the human body. Our bodies work best when we supply them with the proper nutrition God intended. God programmed our bodies to heal themselves—like the natural healing of a cut or sprained ankle.

God gave us glorious bodies that can repair themselves of many ailments if we nourish them well. In turn, *when we are healthy, we can serve God better.* Unfortunately, when tired, foggy brained, or downright ill, we focus on ourselves instead of serving him. If you want to improve the way you feel, *make the decision* to stop eating sugar and refined carbohydrates. This is the first step of the seven-step plan.

If you choose to adopt this lifestyle, you will lose weight, but more importantly, you will improve your health. You won't starve yourself either. Recently, a friend on a cruise told me, "You eat as much as I do. How do you stay slender?" I replied, "The types of food I eat make the difference."

Many times, we do not make positive changes to improve our health until we experience a crisis. For my sister, it was rosacea. While on vacation, she got a rash all over her face. She FaceTimed me and I could see the raised, rough areas of skin. The red bumps came to a head as unsightly pustules. In her high-pitched, stressed voice she asked what I thought it might be. I didn't know, but I suggested she consult her dermatologist as soon as she returned from vacation.

The doctor wasn't sure if it was psoriasis or rosacea. He gave her two creams for her face and an antibiotic to ingest. The creams and antibiotics helped the rash go away, but as soon as she quit taking them, the outbreak came right back. A month later, her dermatologist confirmed the diagnosis of rosacea, which has no cure. Either she stayed on the medications for the rest of her life, or the rosacea reappeared.

She decided to do some research (*acquired* knowledge—step 2) of her own. She discovered sugary foods exacerbate rosacea. When she evaluated what she ate, she realized that sweets and refined carbohydrates made up a large part of her diet. However, she did not like the red, bumpy rash on her face, so she decided to make a change (*decide*—step 1). Throughout this book, we will learn about the steps she took to make a lifestyle change to heal herself of rosacea. If you choose to change your eating habits, your body may heal itself of an ailment too.

MY HEALTH CRISIS

I combated a health crisis at the age of forty-nine. In November that year, I had a crown placed on a tooth. Little did I know how that would mark the beginning of losing my good health. Ultimately, over the next nine months, this tooth abscessed and poisoned my body, resulting in ten different medical diagnoses.

One month after the crown, I began having two menstrual cycles every month. The double periods continued, and eventually, fifteen months later, I had surgery to remove two uterine polyps.

Two months later, I experienced depression and craved chocolate. Do you crave chocolate? Where I used to eat a couple of candy bars per year, now I binged on Ghirardelli chocolate every evening.

In March, I was diagnosed with an ovarian cyst, and two months later, adrenal fatigue. Although exhausted, I had difficulty sleeping. By this point, I should have known something was wrong with my body. Nevertheless, I didn't realize the severity of my physical problems even though as a Christian yoga instructor I taught my clients to be in tune with their bodies.

My doctor prescribed three different adrenal vitamins five times a day for my adrenal fatigue. That's fifteen vitamin pills per day! The physician also prescribed progesterone cream for the ovarian cyst and hormonal imbalance, as I was experiencing perimenopause. That summer I was so exhausted that I could not attend my aunt's funeral because I had no stamina to fly across the country. Even my husband and children did not understand how depleted I felt.

In July I saw flashes of light in my left eye when I quickly turned my head to the left. Two months later I was diagnosed with a hole in my retina. Retinal tears can lead to blindness if the retina becomes detached.

In August, I began experiencing visual migraines even though I had never suffered from headaches. That month I went to my dentist for a cleaning and told my hygienist I felt a bump above one of my teeth. She informed me that was not a good sign, and the dentist discovered the tooth I had crowned in November had abscessed and drained its putrid fluid into my gastrointestinal system. I still didn't realize that the affects of my abscessed tooth likely caused all the other symptoms.

I had an emergency root canal along with ten days of antibiotics and two weeks of steroids. Afterward, I was so fatigued I could not put away the groceries after shopping. No one understood how depleted my system was because on the outside I looked fine, but on the inside, I was a train wreck.

In September my doctor found I was anemic and low in vitamin D, so he told me to take iron and vitamin D supplements. He also referred me to an optometrist for the flashes of light in my eye. The optometrist performed emergency laser surgery to prevent a detached retina. When I turn my head sharply to the left, I still have a flash of light, and I will never regain that part of my vision.

In the fall, my health further declined. I felt utterly drained and sick all the time, and I could have easily stayed in bed. However, my family needed me. My doctors were unable to do much for me except recommend vitamin D, iron supplements, adrenal vitamins, and progesterone cream. So I began alternative health-care therapies such as massage, acupuncture, and colonic irrigation.

Through a colonic irrigation, the therapist found a candida infection in my colon. I had never heard of this type of infection before despite being an RN since candidiasis (candida infection from a Candida fungus) of the gut is not taught in mainstream medicine. Even my internal medicine doctor didn't know how to rid me of this yeast infection in my intestine.

A candida infection in your colon is similar to a vaginal yeast infection. Women are prone to getting vaginal yeast infections when they take antibiotics because the drug kills off beneficial flora in a person's body. Well, I had just consumed antibiotics and a steroid.

I turned fifty that August and lost my health. For fifty years, I took my good health for granted. Now I realized it was precious. Ultimately, what occurred in my body was a poisoning from an abscessed tooth resulting in ten different medical diagnoses in the following order:

1. Bimonthly periods caused by uterine polyps
2. Depression
3. Ovarian cyst
4. Adrenal fatigue
5. Hormonal imbalance
6. Retinal tear
7. Visual migraine
8. Anemia
9. Low vitamin D level
10. Candidiasis infection of my colon

My colonic therapist gave me the book *The Body Ecology Diet* by Donna Gates so I could educate myself. The information in this book confirmed I had an overgrowth of Candida in my gastrointestinal system. I followed the steps outlined in *The Body Ecology Diet* to get rid of the infection.

Candida feeds off of carbohydrates. Therefore, a physical component of my craving for sugar and carbs was an overgrowth of this harmful microorganism. Having candidiasis is like having a monster take control of your appetite. However, I fought this culprit and restored my gut flora. The gut flora consists of beneficial microorganisms (also known as probiotics) that strengthen the immune system and help defend against unfriendly bacteria and pathogens that cause disease.[4]

For the following eight months, I struggled to regain my health. To eradicate the Candida, I continued the regimen from the book and stopped eating fruit, rice, flour, sugar, and desserts. I lost a lot of weight. During this time, I took one step forward and two steps back, then three steps forward and one step back. It was a slow process, but after eight months of being on the strict anti-Candida diet, I finally regained my health.

I felt healed. The diet required great self-control, but I was determined to succeed because I desperately wanted my health back. Ultimately I beat the candida infection in my colon and restored my adrenal glands. God gave us glorious bodies that will heal themselves if we give them the right building blocks.

If you want to determine if you have a candida overgrowth in your gut, take the Candida Quiz at CandiQuiz.com.

MAKE A DECISION ABOUT YOUR HEALTH

Do you want your health back too? You may be experiencing a health crisis and need to make a change. Are you overweight or experiencing problematic symptoms such as depression, moodiness, low energy, achy joints, diabetes, hypertension, or other health problems? Do you crave unhealthy foods? Do you need guidance regarding how to improve your health and lose weight? If you want to make a change, this book will walk you through the process to regain your health through a lifestyle change so you can feel energetic again and begin to live the purposeful and fulfilled life God intended for you.

The first step to getting off sugar and carbohydrates is to decide—decide to make necessary modifications. No one can make this decision for you; it is your choice. However, the next steps will help you maintain your commitment to this life-saving decision. Several other critical components to the process of getting off sugar and carbs include acquiring the right information, obtaining a support system, and praying and asking God to give you the willpower to overcome.

If you accepted Christ as your Savior, you have the Holy Spirit inside you, as 1 Corinthians 6:19–20 states, "Don't you realize that your body is the temple of the Holy Spirit, who lives in you and was given to you by God? You do not belong to yourself, for God bought you with a high price. So you must honor God with your body." When you make healthy eating choices, you take care of the temple God gave you. You only have one body, and it needs to last a lifetime.

Gluttony, which is overeating, is a sin, as implied in Proverbs 23:1–3, "When you sit to dine with a ruler, note well what is before you, and put a knife to your throat if you are given to gluttony. Do not crave his delicacies, for that food is deceptive" (NIV), and Proverbs 23:20–21, "Do not join those who drink too much wine or gorge themselves on meat, for drunkards and gluttons become poor, and drowsiness clothes them in rags" (NIV).

Proverbs 23:1–3 is quite grave when it states, "put a knife to your throat." The truth is, if you overeat like a king, your lifespan shortens. Many chronic diseases such as diabetes and hypertension can be improved, or even cured, by changing eating habits and losing weight. For example, my aunt stopped taking blood pressure medication when she lost ten pounds, because her high blood pressure went away.

The delicacies and deceptive foods mentioned in Proverbs 23:3 are similar to the super-rich and processed foods so accessible today. Neither is nutritious for the body. A person feels awful after consuming them. These delicacies remind me of the desserts I ate on the cruise. During my cruise, I ate like a queen with three-course meals. I tried to eat more fruits and vegetables and lean meats, but I couldn't resist the desserts. After I returned home, it took a month to get my usual energy level back. Being clothed in drowsiness (Proverbs 23:21) accurately describes how people feel after consuming a heavy meal. Sleepiness descends upon them.

Overindulging to our heart's content leads to slavery over the item our flesh desires. This slavery becomes more restrictive than following healthy guidelines. Eating healthy foods gives us the boundaries we need.

FOOD ADDICTION

In our society, the overabundance of delicacies is hard to resist. At first, it seems fun to eat whatever we desire. However, that momentary pleasure is fleeting. It is unhealthy to overeat, and when that becomes a habit, eventually we become addicted to food and can't stop eating. Therefore, we binge.

Regrettably, people become addicted to sugar and carbs. In fact, their brain's circuitry goes haywire when they come into contact with these addictive foods, and their mind assigns supreme value to that food. Magnetic resonance imaging (MRI) of the brain found that addicts' neural circuitry kicks into high gear when the brain lusts for the product of addiction.[5]

Therefore, from a physical perspective, we can become addicted to sugar, wheat, and refined carbohydrates through a biochemical addiction in the brain, or through the cravings caused by Candida, or both. However, we are more than physical beings; we are spiritual as well. The struggle to get off carbs may not be only a physical battle but a spiritual one too. One of the ways we can fight food addiction is through scripture. Appendix 1 includes Bible verses to recite to tap into God's power and strength. If you are addicted to sugar and carbohydrates, like my sister, you will need God's superpower. Paul tells us in Philippians 4:13, "For I can do everything through Christ, who gives me strength."

DIET AFFECTS BRAIN HEALTH

Once you've decided to make this lifestyle change, the dietary changes outlined in step 4 may benefit not only yourself but your family members as well. A diet high in sugar is linked to dementia and Alzheimer's. Scientific studies revealed a low-glycemic, low-carbohydrate diet helps prevent and improve these prevalent, devastating diseases. If you would like more information on how to prevent these diseases, check out my pamphlet "How to Prevent, Improve, and Reverse Alzheimer's and Dementia" go to SusanUNeal.com/ALZ. This pamphlet lists twenty-four interventions to fight these diseases of the brain.

To prevent Alzheimer's and dementia, start interventions early before symptoms begin. If you contract one of these diseases, can someone in your family take care of you? I understand this situation, as my ninety-year-old mother has vascular dementia (from a stroke) and my father-in-law died of Alzheimer's disease.

Brain Testing

Take an online cognitive test to determine the health of your brain. Amazingly, the foods we eat affect our brain function. Access a free online cognitive test, the Self-Administered Gerocognitive Exam (SAGE), at ElderGuru.com. Click on Sage Alzheimer's Exam on the right lower panel.

Cognitive Assessment Results

Write down the results from your cognitive assessments here.

MAKE YOUR COMMITMENT

Now that you have decided to take this seven-step plan to improving your health and your future, the following actions will help you stay accountable to your commitment and give you a baseline to measure against once you have made progress on your journey to wholeness.

Contract

Take the first step to get off sugar and carbohydrates by deciding to make a lifestyle change. Begin by writing a contract between you and God on the lines below. Include the measurable goals you would like to achieve. Ask God to help you and place your success in his loving hands.

. . .

_____

_____

_____

Baseline Assessment

Now that you have decided to conquer sugar and carbs, you'll need to take a few measurements before moving on. First, before changing your eating habits, obtain a baseline of your current condition. Weigh yourself and measure your waistline.

Date to implement changes:

Baseline measurement date:

Weight:

Waistline:

Symptom Checklist

Put a check by the following unhealthy symptoms you experience.

_____ Fatigue

_____ Anxiety

_____ Insomnia

_____ Irritability

_____ Depression

_____ Mood swings

_____ Poor memory

_____ Food allergies

_____ Foggy brained

_____ Decreased sex drive

_____ Hormonal imbalance

_____ Chronic fatigue, fibromyalgia

_____ Vaginal yeast infections, urinary tract infections

_____ Craving sweets and refined carbohydrates or alcohol

_____ Digestive issues (bloating, constipation, diarrhea) or disorders

_____ Skin and nail infections such as toenail fungus, athlete's foot, and ringworm

Dietary Assessment

Record the foods you ate last week. Recalling these foods will test your memory as well as help you realize the kind of foods you typically consume. How well does your memory recall? Do wheat and sugar comprise a large part of your diet?

_____

_____

_____

_____

. . .

After six months of changing your eating habits, you will objectively measure your cognitive abilities by retaking the online cognitive test, recheck your weight and waistline measurements, and note whether any unhealthy symptoms subsided. A reassessment survey is provided at the end of step 7.

TAKING STEP 1: DECIDE

Making the decision to commit to a lifestyle change, particularly if you struggle with food addiction is crucial. While it may be difficult to commit, once you have, you can look back on your contract with God when things get tough. Remember, no matter if and when you make a mistake, you can get back on track. Each chapter will end with a list of action steps to help you accomplish that step. In step 1, complete the following action steps:

1. If you haven't already, watch the Ted-Ed video, "How Does Sugar Affect the Brain?" by the neuroscientist Nicole Avena, Ph.D. Go to ScienceAlert.com/watch-this-is-how-sugar-affects-your-brain.
2. Check labels to make sure you don't consume sugary foods with greater than ten grams of sugar per serving.
3. Write and sign your contract between you and God.
4. Complete your assessments.

7 Steps to Get Off Sugar and Carbohydrates:
   STEP 1: Decide to improve your health through proper nutrition.

STEP 2: ACQUIRE A SUPPORT SYSTEM AND KNOWLEDGE

Decide—>**Acquire**—>Clean Out—>Purchase—>Plan—>Prepare—>Improve

A decision to change one's lifestyle can't be maintained without support. The next step in the journey is to acquire that support—to gain the knowledge to make necessary changes and create a system for encouragement and accountability. We are comprised of a body, mind, and spirit, so all the components of our well-being must be addressed to successfully make the changes needed to improve our health. You will learn about food addiction and Candida (physical), which foods are beneficial versus harmful (intellectual), the benefit of obtaining a support system (emotional), and memorizing Bible verses (spiritual).

ACQUIRE KNOWLEDGE

Gaining knowledge regarding unhealthy versus healthy foods is crucial to making this lifestyle change. You cannot keep your new commitment without understanding how and why to take the next steps. Resources in this chapter will educate and equip you for this journey. Making a lifestyle change to improve your health will be challenging, including physical (biochemical), emotional, and spiritual trials. In step 2, you acquire strategies to address these challenges.

Understanding Food Addiction

We need to understand that sugar and wheat are addictive. Addiction is a compulsive repetition of an activity despite life-damaging consequences. Food addiction is a biochemical disorder that cannot be controlled by willpower alone. If you have not considered the possibility of having a food addiction, do not feel shame over the terminology. Your body has fallen prey to the accumulative effects of sugar and wheat that are ingrained in so many of our culture's food habits. The surgeon general's 2016 report indicated that addiction is a chronic brain disease, not a moral failing.[1]

Two hallmarks of addiction include persistent desire and repeated unsuccessful attempts to stop. Being addicted to food is like having an alien inside of you who takes control of your body and eats a bunch of unhealthy food. You can't stop it. Sugar and wheat hijack your body. You can't halt the craving or binges no matter what diet or method you try. Your own willpower is never enough. Understanding that food addiction is not a lack of self-control, but a rewiring of the brain, helps you to be more compassionate with yourself.

How does this addiction happen? Foods containing sugar and wheat cause the release of an excess amount of dopamine in the brain. Dopamine, a feel-good neurohormone, releases when we eat foods high in sugar, take opiate drugs, smoke cigarettes, drink alcohol, cuddle with our kids, pet a dog, or enjoy sex.[2] A dopamine rush can rewire the brain to desire more of whatever causes its release. Therefore, when a food addict sees sugary foods, dopamine releases and causes the person's focus to narrow.[3] She can think only about eating that food item to experience the euphoria it brings.

Scientists found that the part of the brain that restrains behavior (self-control) was abnormally quiet in rats with an addiction. Unfortunately, when we struggle with the desire for unhealthy foods, the part of the brain that inhibits addictive behavior becomes silent, and we lose the ability to have self-control.[4] Sugar and refined carbohydrates take over and restructure the brain.

In 2017, scientists conducted trials of a new therapy for addicts called transcranial magnetic stimulation (TMS), which treated depression and migraines for years. TMS runs an electric current through a wand that alters the electrical activity in the brain to activate the drug-damaged neural pathways that restrain behavior. So far the therapy is successful.[5] If studies continue to be successful, this could be a life-changing option for people addicted to a variety of substances.

In addition to being addictive, sugar and refined carbohydrates cause disease. Chronic ailments such as diabetes, high blood pressure, and obesity are related to the consumption of too much of the wrong types of food. Therefore, gaining knowledge is essential to changing one's eating habits.

Determining whether you are a food addict will help you understand yourself and enable you to effectively overcome this addiction. Use these online quizzes to determine if you are addicted to food: FoodAddicts.org/am-i-a-food-addict or OA.org/newcomers/how-do-i-start/are-you-a-compulsive-overeater/.

If you have an emotional connection with food, please consider using the *Christian Study Guide for 7 Steps to Get Off Sugar and Carbohydrates*. Whether you do this study by yourself or with a group, it will help you go more in-depth to resolve an emotional issue once and for all.

In my course, 7 Steps to Reclaim Your Health and Optimal Weight (https://susanuneal.com/courses/7-steps-to-get-off-sugar-and-carbs-course), I help you figure out and resolve the root cause of your inappropriate eating habit. One solved, taming your appetite is much easier. I show you how to change your eating habits once and for all.

If you are a food addict, I recommend you join a Christian-based weight-loss program or a twelve-step food addiction program along with a corresponding support group. Appendix 2 provides a resource list for these groups. Some Christian programs include:

First Place 4 Health (FirstPlace4Health.com) offers a biblical approach to weight loss through a series of Bible studies. Online groups are available, or you can check to see if one exists in your area.

Take Back Your Temple (TakeBackYourTemple.com) is a Christian online weight loss program whose motto is "Your body for God's glory. We help you take back your house so you can fulfill your God-given purpose."

The Eden Diet: A Biblical and Merciful Anti-Dieting Plan for Weight Loss (TheEdenDiet.com), a Christian weight-loss program with online support groups.

Thin Within: A Non-Diet Grace Based Approach (ThinWithin.org) is a Christian weight management program that includes online classes and groups.

Barb Raveling Christian weight loss products (Barb Raveling.com). include, a podcast—Taste for Truth: Christian Weight Loss, an app—I Deserve a Donut: and Other Lies That Make You Eat, and a couple of books—*Taste for Truth: A 30 Day Weight Loss Bible Study* and *I Deserve a Donut: And Other Lies that Make You Eat.*

Grace Filled Plate (GraceFilledPlate.com) is a website with an excellent blog which includes having a healthy mindset, recipes, nutrition, and faith.

Victory Steps for Women: Christian Weight Loss & Spiritual Wellness (VictorySteps.net/christian-weight-loss-program.html), a faith-based health and wellness coaching program, helps women overcome emotional eating, binge eating, and compulsive overeating behaviors.

Weight Loss, God's Way (CathyMorenzie.com/challenge/) is a Christian-based weight loss program that offers a free twenty-one-day challenge.

Three different online food addiction programs include:
OA.org/ (OA is Overeater's Anonymous)
FoodAddicts.org/

FoodAddictsanonymous.org/

Joining an online support group is another way to share the ups and downs of this journey. Connecting with like-minded individuals who are persevering through the same trials as you helps divide the load. Through these support groups, you can exchange acquired knowledge about your shared journey. In addition, sometimes we need to vent and express our disappointment or success with another person who understands. Life sharing nourishes the emotional side of our well-being.

Understanding Candida

Candida is the second potential physical component to a compulsion to overeat refined carbohydrates. If you crave sugar, alcohol, and processed foods, you might have an imbalance in the flora of your gut. An imbalance means the beneficial microorganisms (probiotics) have been killed off by antibiotics, steroids, unhealthy processed foods, and chemicals in foods. The destruction of these beneficial microbes allows the harmful microbe Candida to multiply quickly, taking over your digestive tract. Candida Albicans, a type of yeast common in the gut, can grow roots into the lining of your gastrointestinal (GI) system. The fungal overgrowth creates openings in the bowel walls, which is known as a leaky gut. These holes allow harmful microorganisms to enter the bloodstream. Our bodies don't recognize these particles, so our immune system creates antibodies which cause food allergies and autoimmune diseases to develop.[6] An overgrowth of Candida also causes your abdomen to become distended.

When Candida spreads out of control, it acts like a parasite sucking the life and energy out of you. Candida feeds on carbs, which is why you crave them. It is like a monster growing inside of you, craving sugar, and it is hard to fight its never-ending appetite.

I had an overgrowth of Candida in my colon, so I know how hard it is to fight this culprit. Yet I wanted my health back, so I struggled to restore my health through an anti-Candida cleanse, which I will discuss in step 4. It took eight months on a rigorous non-Candida diet to regain my health, but with determination, by the power of the Holy Spirit, I succeeded.

Below is a list of symptoms that might arise from an overgrowth of Candida. This survey is the same list you completed in step 1. Check off the ones that apply to you now. The more symptoms you experience, the more likely you are to have a candida infection.

_____ Fatigue

_____ Anxiety

_____ Insomnia

_____ Irritability

_____ Depression

_____ Mood swings

_____ Poor memory

_____ Food allergies

_____ Foggy brained

_____ Decreased sex drive

_____ Hormonal imbalance

_____ Chronic fatigue, fibromyalgia

_____ Vaginal yeast infections, urinary tract infections

_____ Craving sweets and refined carbohydrates or alcohol

_____ Digestive issues (bloating, constipation, diarrhea) or disorders

_____ Skin and nail infections such as toenail fungus, athlete's foot, and ringworm

All of the symptoms listed above are indicative of a Candida infection in your gut. If you previously took an antibiotic, you might have an imbalance of the flora in your GI tract because antibiotics kill off the beneficial microorganisms, which allows the yeast to multiply rapidly. The more times in your life that you have taken antibiotics, without replenishing your gut with probiotics that contain greater than ten strains of microorganisms for several weeks, the more likely you have candidiasis.

A simple spit test can determine if you have an overgrowth of

Candida. First thing in the morning, before you drink anything or brush your teeth, spit into a glass of water. In one to three minutes, check the cup to see if any strings hang from the spit—strings are a positive sign of Candida. The spit will resemble a jellyfish. If the water becomes cloudy or the saliva sinks to the bottom, this is also a positive sign. Healthy saliva floats on the top of the water with no strings hanging down.

There are two websites that provide a detailed explanation of the spit test. The first is NationalCandidaCenter.com. Click on the Tests tab at the top. From the menu that appears, click on Self-Test 2 - My Body Fluids.The second website is CandidaSupport.org/resources/saliva-test/. These two websites also include written Candida tests you can complete for further assessment.

Candida will take over your life if left untreated. If you exhibit many of the numerous symptoms listed above, you need to restore the balance of microorganisms in your gastrointestinal system. An excellent resource to help you learn more about restoring your intestinal flora is *The Body Ecology Diet* by Donna Gates. Check out her website BodyEcology.com/. Her follow-up book, *The Body Ecology Guide to Growing Younger*, is another excellent resource.

Harmful Versus Beneficial Foods

Realizing a slice of bread will raise your blood-sugar level higher than sugar should motivate you not to eat bread. Begin to learn which foods are damaging versus beneficial—the ones God gave us to eat, not the food industry's offerings.

Today, grocery stores and restaurants make non-gluten food choices readily available. Why has gluten sensitivity skyrocketed in the US? Fifty years ago, sensitivity to gluten was rare. I believe it is because the human body cannot proficiently digest the gluten in wheat the way it is hybridized now.

For centuries, people flourished by consuming bread. Nevertheless, the problem with wheat is that it is not the same today as it was one hundred years ago. Norman Borlaug received the Nobel Peace

Prize in 1970 in recognition of his contributions to world peace through increasing the food supply through hybridization—cross-breeding of different varieties—of wheat.[7]

He crossbred various types of wheat to create a high-yield dwarf wheat. No longer do tall amber waves of grain grow in the Midwest. Instead, wheat is now only a couple of feet tall, drought resistant, and prolific. *Unfortunately, the gluten changed so much that it can induce gluten sensitivity.*[8] Therefore, do not consume any wheat products. No waffles, pancakes, muffins, cake, piecrust, pizza, pretzels, bread, pasta —the list goes on and on.

Since gluten in the hybridized wheat is difficult to digest, some individuals become sensitive or intolerant to the gluten.[9] These individuals experience digestive problems when they consume foods with gluten (wheat, rye, and barley). When my sister consumes gluten, she needs to be close to a bathroom for the next twenty-four hours. Her gluten sensitivity blood test (tTG-IgA and IgG) confirmed her sensitivity to gluten.

However, gluten sensitivity tests are not always accurate. Another member of my family who is gluten sensitive had the same test with negative results. My doctor confirmed the high incidence of false-negative gluten-sensitivity test results. Instead, he recommended an individual remove wheat and gluten from their diet for a month to determine how sensitive the body might be to these foods.

If you want to find out if you are gluten sensitive, either take the Gluten Quiz at GlutenIntoleranceQuiz.com, or fast from gluten for a whole month. This length of time is necessary because the gluten molecule is so large it may take weeks before the body can eliminate it. As you reintroduce gluten back into your diet, note any adverse side effects such as gas, bloating, diarrhea, smelly feces, constipation, abdominal pain, nausea, vomiting, foggy mind, headache, joint pain, depression, nasal congestion, skin problems, fatigue, and autoimmune diseases. If you experience any of these symptoms, gluten from wheat is food you should not consume.

If a person's body does not recognize gluten as food, their immune system attacks the gluten and, unfortunately, their body at the same time. The intestinal lining becomes damaged, resulting in holes in the intestinal wall (called leaky gut). Those holes allow food to enter the bloodstream.[10] In turn, a person may become allergic to other types of food as well. It is not surprising that gluten sensitivity is often paired with an autoimmune condition because the body accidentally starts harming its own cells as it attacks the broken-down food particles in the bloodstream.

Gluten is in wheat, barley, and rye. Yet breads made of barley and rye are uncommon. Therefore, I believe the gluten culprit comes from the hybridization of wheat. Remember, a polypeptide from wheat passes through the blood-brain barrier and goes to the opiate receptors in the brain. This likely contributes to a rise of autoimmune diseases in the US.

In other words, if you get an autoimmune disease, it could have been caused by a gluten sensitivity you didn't know you had. This sensitivity could have caused your immune system to get confused and attack a part of your body. Therefore, I recommend anyone with an autoimmune disease not eat wheat.

Most Americans have no idea wheat has been bred to the point the body thinks of it as a foreign substance. This is from hybridization. But what if the body doesn't recognize genetically modified food? Again, a person's immune system might attack the foreign substance and its own body at the same time. Consequently, you should avoid any GMO foods. The only way to do so is to purchase organic foods.

The United States is one of the few industrialized nations in the world that does not label GMO food products. Finally, in July 2016 a bill passed that requires GMO food labeling within two years. The food industries fought the GMO labeling for years to avoid decreased sales or the need to change the composition of their ingredients.

Unfortunately, food manufacturers picked up on the gluten-free trend and created all sorts of unhealthy, nongluten products. Substituting wheat with gluten-free processed foods is not a healthy alternative, since they often contain rice flour, which raises blood-sugar levels.

High blood-sugar levels cause a person's pancreas to release insulin. Increased insulin causes the body to store belly fat.[11] Do you have belly fat? What you eat plays a huge role in gaining fat around the middle. High blood-sugar levels from the wrong foods lead to insulin resistance, type-2 diabetes, and dementia. In fact, dementia is referred to as type-3 diabetes—which is on the rise from consuming too much sugar and processed foods. That is why I asked you to complete the online cognitive assessment in step 1.

Delicious unhealthy foods are conveniently available to us. But just because we have access to them and the freedom to eat them doesn't mean we should. If we understand which products are harmful, we can avoid them. You may have had no idea that wheat was harmful until reading this book. However, gaining accurate knowledge about food is not always easy because of the amount of either false or conflicting information available. Be discerning as you acquire food knowledge and ensure it is from a reputable source.

If you can't or don't want to eliminate bread from your diet, make homemade gluten-free bread to avoid wheat. My sister uses the recipe Kim's Gluten Free, Dairy Free, Whole Grain Bread at GFReal-Food.com (see the last recipe in appendix 4). You could also obtain a freshly ground flour made from a nonhybridized whole-wheat berry (not just part of the berry). Einkorn wheat, a variety of nonhybridized wheat, might be available from a local provider that stone grinds the whole kernel into whole-grain einkorn flour. I found such a supplier at a local farmer's market in Pensacola, Florida. Her business is Our Daily Bread, and the Facebook page is Facebook.com/ourdailybread-bakerypensacola/. I purchase freshly ground whole grain einkorn flour from her.

To slowly wean my family off of processed white flour, I started by making pancakes, waffles, muffins, and other baked goods with 1/2 einkorn and 1/2 white flour. Surprisingly, they acclimated well to this half-and-half mixture. Then I increased the einkorn flour to 3/4 with 1/4 white flour—I got some negative feedback about this, but they got used to it (my family preferred the 50/50 combination).

My baked goods were denser but still delicious. If I made recipes with 100 percent einkorn flour, my family would not eat much of it.

So I had to settle for using 3/4 einkorn flour. With a family, making this lifestyle change can be tough, as it is hard to please everyone. Providing healthy alternatives your family will eat can be challenging.

I explained to my family that I needed to make these dietary changes to get my health back. I wanted to feel energetic again, and they desired this too—since they benefited when I felt well. (When Mama ain't happy, ain't nobody happy.) Their understanding helped them go along with my dietary changes as much as their taste buds could tolerate.

For me, I could not eat baked goods with any white flour. My gut had been too damaged when I was ill. If I eat these delicious baked products, I wake up feeling tired and foggy brained. After being weaned off unhealthy foods, I can tell when one food item affects me negatively.

With time, you should become more aware of how different foods affect how you feel. This correlation will become apparent as you keep a record of what you eat and how it makes you feel in your journal (appendix 3; we will discuss journaling later in this chapter). After a while, a pattern may emerge. If I eat something that raises my blood-sugar level, I do not feel good the next day. How do you feel the day after consuming food with high sugar content?

Roundup Ready Crops

These crops are genetically engineered to be resistant to the carcinogen glyphosate, which is the primary ingredient in the herbicide Roundup.[12] Farmers who produce Roundup Ready crops are free to spray Roundup on their fields throughout the growing season, as the plants are resistant to this herbicide. In the United States most of the nation's corn, wheat, oats, soy, and sugar beets are Roundup Ready crops.[13] Can you imagine what this carcinogen may do to the beneficial bacteria in your gut or to your overall health? Therefore, you should only eat these foods if they are organic. Organic foods are not GMO or Roundup Ready crops.

. . .

Unhealthy Food Combinations

A friend told me she experienced painful heartburn after eating salmon, brussel sprouts, and a baked potato. She didn't know why she felt so terrible since these were healthy foods. She didn't understand what happens during digestion with different food combinations.

I explained how some food combinations cause indigestion. Combining a protein with a baked potato may cause heartburn. Conversely, eating a protein with vegetables does not cause indigestion, nor does eating a baked potato with vegetables. It's the protein/potato combination that doesn't digest well together.[14]

Also, eating fruit with your meal is not a suitable combination because fruit digests quickly, but other foods, such as proteins, do not. Therefore, eat fruit alone and wait twenty to thirty minutes before eating anything else. *The Body Ecology Diet* by Donna Gates includes a great section about food combinations and which ones cause indigestion.

Food Triggers

Another critical component to the physical nature of food addiction is understanding food triggers. Triggers cause us to get right back on the merry-go-round of desire, binging, and withdrawal. Identify your food triggers—the aroma of freshly baked cookies, a dessert table at a restaurant, a food commercial, or even an emotion. Choose to get off that merry-go-round by recognizing what stimuli set you off and avoid them. Turn the channel or pick up something to read. Call your accountability partner or recite a Bible verse. Seek help from an online support group.

Unfortunately, if you are a food addict you have to consider yourself as a recovering addict who has quit your drug—wheat and sugar. Therefore, you cannot consume these products ever again, or you will go right back to being addicted to them and having the undesirable symptoms that accompany their consumption. Yet you can live a full life without consuming these delicious but detrimental products.

ACQUIRE A SUPPORT SYSTEM

Obtaining a support system helps address the emotional aspect of this transformation. As Ecclesiastes 4:12 tells us, "Though one may be overpowered, two can defend themselves. A cord of three strands is not quickly broken" (NIV). I recommend that in addition to online or live support groups, you ask someone to be your accountability and prayer partner.

It is validating when someone understands how we feel. Perhaps no one in your family understands your struggle, so it is helpful to reach out to others. Also, family can sometimes enable our bad habits because they don't really understand, or they're in the same boat, but because you're so close you give each other permission to stay on the bad habit pathway. Having a friend for accountability who you can call when temptation arises is a crucial key to your success. It is powerful when a friend speaks the truth in love. Pray with your friend. The security of knowing someone prays for you is comforting.

At times all of us eat unhealthy foods. When this happens, we may experience guilt and depression. Having someone to pray for us during these challenges is essential to our spiritual victory. In fact, calling a friend when we feel temptation can redirect our thought process from the food. You could ask your friend to pray with you or you could meet at a coffee shop to get away from the temptation. Be open and express what's causing a challenge for you.

My sister shared the challenges she faced while she changed her eating habits. She got hungry in the afternoons, and finding a healthy snack remained difficult. I gave her suggestions and prayed with her. She decided to move her family's dinner time earlier so she could satisfy her hunger. Sharing trials with a friend helps diffuse the burden. I prayed for her and with her many times during her transitory journey.

The following scripture confirms we should share trials and confess our sins to one another: "Confess your sins to each other and pray for each other so that you may be healed. The earnest prayer of a righteous person has great power and produces wonderful results"

(James 5:16). Bringing our struggles out of the closet, and sharing them with someone we trust is valuable. Prayers are powerful, especially from someone who loves and understands us for who we truly are—including the good, the bad, and the ugly.

For additional support, please join my closed Facebook group, 7 Steps to Get Off Sugar and Carbohydrates, and share with me how you are doing.

Journal

Record your path to recovery in a journal. Writing down your actual food choices each day, as well as your thoughts, feelings, struggles, and victories, has a powerful effect. Journaling will create personal accountability. The more you journal, the more easily you'll recognize when you are eating out of emotion or for the wrong reasons. You will see what helped you battle the struggles previously. Journaling will provide clarity of your thoughts, feelings, and desires.

To help you with journaling, I created the *Healthy Living Journal*. It is full of charts and each day you'll record water and food intake, exercise, energy level, and corresponding moods. Recording your daily food consumption provides an opportunity to learn how food affects your health. When you discover negative health patterns you can change. Devotions and educational snippets are provided on a daily basis too.

If you want to create your own journal, the following information should be included in the journal (see appendix 3). Write the following items in your journal:

1. The time you eat.
2. Why you want to eat. Are you hungry, bored, angry? Is it just "time to eat" or are you with others who are having a meal?
3. If you feel a strong emotion related to this consumption of food, record the emotion.

4. Food you ate and drank, including quantity.
5. How you feel after you ate? Are you satisfied or stuffed?
6. Energy level and clarity of mind after you ate.
7. When waking up in the morning, how do you feel? See if there is a pattern of eating high-sugar-content foods and feeling sluggish the next morning.
8. What are you grateful for today?
9. Prayer requests to God.
10. Exercise—type of activity and length of time.
11. Number of glasses of water you drank and when. Did you drink on an empty stomach?
12. Every time you binge, record: what you ate, why you ate it, what triggered you to eat it, and what you might do the next time you are tempted.

As you write this information, recognize any patterns between your emotions and food consumption. Do you eat because you were hungry? If not, why? Did at least three hours lapse between meals? It takes three to four hours before food digests and your stomach empties.

You can journal on paper or electronically, on your phone or computer. The My Fitness Pal phone app is an excellent resource to track food, calories, and activity level.

If you recognize that you have a dysfunctional relationship with food, when did this dysfunction begin? The more extended the period, the longer it will take to reset your body and mind. Changing your eating habits is not an overnight process. But step-by-step you can reprogram your body, mind, and spirit. Creating a support system and journaling are vital components to your success.

Scripture

Another essential component of this lifestyle change is tapping into God's power through reciting Bible verses. God's Word offers guidance to every area of life, including our health and our emotions. Since emotions trigger negative food habits, learn to use this weapon as you need it. Appendix 1 includes a list of scriptures categorized by the emotion a person experiences. Speak these verses out loud and with authority, believing in their power. The spoken Word of God is a double-edged sword that defeats the enemy.

Advantages of memorizing scripture include reducing stress, resisting temptation, hearing God speak, and receiving comforting reassurance of God's steadfast love. There are several steps to learning Bible verses.[15] First, you need motivation. Without God-given inspiration, memorization is difficult. So pray and ask God for the desire. For years, I thought I couldn't learn verses because they were too challenging to remember. However, with prayer and God's help, the Holy Spirit empowered me to memorize numerous scriptures.

Next, which scriptures should you memorize? Sometimes while doing a Bible study or reading the Bible, the Holy Spirit led me to learn a specific verse. A verse may be important personally. For example, as I was raising young children, verses on how to discipline children were relevant for me to memorize at the time. What are you currently going through? Seek the verses that apply to your current life situation and challenge. Many of these are listed in appendix 3, but you will find others as you search the Bible.

The second step to memorizing scripture is to write the Bible verse on an index card in the following manner: Write the verse name and number at the top and bottom of the card. Then, break the verse up into short segments that are easy to memorize. For example:

Philippians 4:13
For I can do everything
through Christ,
who gives me strength.
Philippians 4:13

This simple and effective method makes it easy to learn one line of the verse at a time. Continue to do this until the entire verse is memorized. For me, it was harder to remember the verse name and number than the verse itself. Therefore, I wrote the verse name and number at the top and the bottom of the card.

Review the Bible verse on a weekly basis to remember it. I studied the scripture cards while I worked out at the gym. My husband thought this was a creative way to exercise my body, mind, and spirit through the Word of God. This weekly repetition kept the verses at the forefront of my mind.

Bring the scripture cards with you on a walk, tape one to the bathroom mirror, or keep them in your purse to review. Be creative! Storing God's Word in your heart is like storing up treasure, as indicated in Proverbs 2:6, "For the Lord grants wisdom! His every word is a treasure of knowledge and understanding" (TLB).

If you memorize scripture, you can unsheathe the sword of the Spirit and slash the enemy when he tempts. Hiding God's Word in your heart is vital to your spiritual success on this journey to change.

Prayer

To make the lifestyle changes necessary to improve our health we need to access our heavenly father through prayer. When Jesus was in the garden of Gethsemane sweating blood, he was on his knees praying to his father. We need to follow Jesus's example. God wants to communicate with us, and that's another way we receive his power to face our struggles. Jesus's brother told us in James 5:16, "The earnest prayer of a righteous man has great power and wonderful results" (TLB).

An essential component of the arsenal God gave us is prayer, as Paul indicated in Ephesians 6:18, "And pray in the Spirit on all occasions with all kinds of prayers and requests" (NIV). Prayer helps break down the resistance you may experience as you make these changes.

During prayer, ask God to give you a willing spirit to surrender to him, and replace your desire for food with the desire to please and serve him. Also, incorporate Bible verses into your prayers. For example, "Lord, one may be overpowered, but two can defend themselves (Ecclesiastes 3:12), so please help me to find the perfect prayer partner."

God loves you, and he wants you to succeed. Use his powerful weapons—Bible verses and prayer.

Other Resources

Neurologist David Perlmutter MD wrote the book *Grain Brain: The Surprising Truth About Wheat, Carbs, and Sugar—Your Brain's Silent Killers*. He recommends taking a probiotic that contains at least ten billion active cultures from at least ten different strains of beneficial bacteria to help fight the overgrowth of Candida and balance your gut flora. As this book's subtitle (*Your Brain's Silent Killers*) indicates— wheat, sugar, and carbs harm the human brain.

The Daniel Plan by Rick Warren, recommends you stop eating sugar, wheat, and milk products for one week. Then reintroduce one of those foods at a time back into your diet to determine any adverse effects.

If you have a food addiction or emotional connection with food, please consider using the *Christian Study Guide for 7 Steps to Get Off Sugar and Carbohydrates.*

I also found *Eat Right 4 Your Type* by Dr. Peter D'Adamo to be helpful in figuring out the foods to avoid to eliminate digestive issues. This book bases food choices on a person's blood type. It recommended that those with my AB blood type not eat sunflower or sesame seeds. Normally I added those seeds to my homemade granola. Yet I often belched after I ate the granola. When I eliminated those seeds from the recipe, my indigestion ceased.

It is vital to notice how your body reacts to certain foods. If you experience digestive problems, keep track of what you ate before the symptom—in your journal. Note whether the food was consistently wheat or dairy. These two products are the usual offenders.

Dr. William Davis, the author of *Wheat Belly*, states, "Whole wheat bread increases blood-sugar as much as or more than sugar." As a cardiologist, he placed his overweight, diabetic-prone patients on a low-glycemic, whole-foods diet that excluded wheat for three months.[16] Results included:

- diabetics became nondiabetic
- acid reflux disappeared
- irritable bowel syndrome went away
- rheumatoid arthritis pain decreased
- asthma symptoms improved or resolved completely
- rashes disappeared
- energy increased
- lost weight
- experienced clearer thinking and greater focus

If you have cancer, diabetes, or a life-threatening disease I recommend trying the Hallelujah Diet at MyHDiet.com/what-is-the-hallelujah-diet/. This biblically based diet does not condone eating meat, only the types of food God gave us in the garden of Eden from Genesis 1:29.

Recipes

We need wholesome recipes that do not include wheat, sugar, white rice, or processed foods. Appendix 4 includes my favorite recipes.

The Daniel Plan: 40 Days to a Healthier Life by Rick Warren, Daniel Amen MD, and Mark Hyman MD includes meal plans with precisely what to eat for each meal as well some recipes. *The Daniel Plan Cookbook* is chock-full of healthy recipes.

Grain Brain book by David Perlmutter MD also contains beneficial recipes.

The Body Ecology Diet by Donna Gates contains tasty, nutritious recipes. Her cookbook *Living Cookbook: Deliciously Healing Foods for a Happier, Healthier World* contains delicious recipes.

Pinterest posts thousands of recipes, but not all may be good for you. You can check out the recipes I selected at Pinterest.com/SusanUNeal/.

TAKING STEP 2: ACQUIRE

Are you interested in learning more about how to become a healthier person? You are well on your way. These are the suggested action steps from this chapter:

1. Take the food addiction test.
2. Join a Christian weight loss or food addiction program.
3. Conduct the Candida spit test.
4. Either take the Gluten Quiz at GlutenIntoleranceQuiz.com, or eliminate wheat for one month, then reintroduce it into to your diet to see if you experience any ill effects.
5. Choose an accountability/prayer partner.
6. Join my closed Facebook group, 7 Steps to Get Off Sugar and Carbohydrates, at Facebook.com/groups/184355458927013/ to gain additional support.
7. Purchase the *Healthy Living Journal* or create your own journal and start recording the items listed in appendix 3.
8. Choose a scripture verse to fight temptation and write it on an index card.

7 Steps to Get Off Sugar and Carbohydrates:
  STEP 1. Decide to improve your health through proper nutrition.
  STEP 2. Acquire a support system and knowledge to help make a lifestyle change.

3

STEP 3: CLEAN OUT THE PANTRY AND REFRIGERATOR

Decide—>Acquire—>**Clean Out**—>Purchase—>Plan—>Prepare—>Improve

Now that you decided to change your eating habits and acquired information about damaging foods, it is time to *clean out* the pantry and refrigerator. It is necessary to remove unhealthy foods, so you are not tempted to eat them. You may need to call on your support system for the willpower and accountability to take this step.

Why do you have to remove everything unhealthy? Remember, triggers, such as a package of cookies, can cause a relapse. Just looking at the bag releases dopamine and an overwhelming desire to consume that unhealthy food.[1] Therefore, you must get these items out of the house. If a family member wants to eat foods that may tempt you, they should keep these packages hidden in their room and out of the pantry. Ask them to honor your goals and help you in this way.

Remember, think of foods as being dead or alive. *Food from a bag sitting on the shelf for months is dead and does not give your body any of the nutrients it needs to be healthy.* A fresh piece of fruit contains essential vitamins, minerals, and fiber that a body needs.

Fiber in fruit and vegetables fills your stomach and tells your body you are full. When the fiber is removed from processed foods, it takes a larger quantity of food to become full. Also, the fiber in fruit slows digestion, which reduces the effects of sugar in raising your blood-sugar levels. As you eliminate processed foods from you diet you should consume more whole, organic fruits, vegetables, whole grains (oats, brown rice, quinoa, barley), beans, fish, and meat. (We will discuss the right foods to purchase in step 4.) Your body will thank you for nourishing it properly and respond by healing.

When I was sick, it was essential to nourish myself with healthy foods so my body could create new, properly functioning cells. I wanted to get well, so I began to evaluate everything I ate.

Today, I look at any food and assess whether or not it is good for me. If a person primarily eats dead food, how does the body get the proper nutrients it needs? If a cell within the human body replicates incorrectly, it is called cancer. How can your body replace old cells with healthy new ones if you don't give it the essential vitamins and minerals it requires?

We need to consume foods similar to what God gave us in the garden of Eden. For example, green beans sautéed in olive oil is healthier than a green bean casserole with mushroom soup and processed onion rings. The casserole is not as healthy for your body as the sautéed green beans.

Check labels and try not to eat foods with more than five ingredients or 10 grams of sugar per serving. The American Heart Association recommends you limit your calories from sugar to no more than half of your total calories, which is a lot. For most women in the US that should be no more than 24 grams of sugar or 100 calories per day. For men it is 36 grams of sugar or 150 calories from sugar per day.

If you can't pronounce an ingredient, your body probably won't recognize it as food either. Begin to simplify the foods you consume. For example, eat two hard-boiled eggs for breakfast, a whole avocado for lunch, and an apple for a snack. Ask yourself, "Did the food I am about to eat exist in the garden of Eden?" Food doesn't have to be complicated.

It wasn't complicated for Adam and Eve. They picked a piece of fruit or a vegetable and ate it. It doesn't have to be difficult for us either. Instead of making an elaborate meal, eat fresh, raw vegetables, which cost less and are better for you than processed, sugar-laden products.

Farmer's markets are great venues to find fresh, local produce. It is best to eat locally grown fruit and vegetables. Buy a potato and bake it with the following toppings: olive oil, broccoli, scallions, and sea salt with kelp. The baked potato is better for you than a bag of potato chips. *Eat foods closer to the form they were in when they came out of the garden.*

FOODS TO ELIMINATE

Understanding what foods are beneficial versus which are harmful is really confusing today, especially since the food industry entices us through great marketing and by adding addictive ingredients. In step 2, we acquired knowledge about food addiction, Candida, and the importance of an accountability and prayer partner. Step 3 will continue this education by providing you with a list of unhealthy foods and the reasons why they do not nourish the human body. It is far better to eat foods as close to their value at harvest—the way God made them—rather than processed foods.

Wheat

As discussed in step 2, I do not recommend eating any foods containing wheat because today's wheat is hybridized, and therefore, is not the same healthy grain that nourished humans for centuries. The gluten in today's dwarf, drought-resistance wheat is extremely difficult for a person to digest.[2] I believe this new form of wheat created in the 1950s caused the high level of gluten sensitivity we see today.

White Flour

Eliminate wheat because it is addictive and the human body has difficulty digesting the gluten. White flour is one of the most prevalent wheat products used today, and it is far removed from the grain it once was. A wheat berry consists of three layers: bran, germ, and endosperm. White flour contains one part of the wheat kernel—the endosperm, which is mostly starch. The other two parts of the wheat contain the *fiber* and *nutrients*, and these *are not included in white flour*. The flour has also been chemically bleached, consequently, the grain no longer resembles the wholesome food God intended.

Before 1870, wheat was stone-ground, and the whole grain was mashed (all three parts of the kernel). The invention of the steel roller revolutionized grain milling. With this device, the components of the wheat berry could be separated. Removing the bran (fiber) and germ (nutrients) significantly extended the shelf life of the processed flour. Stone-ground flour contained natural oils from the wheat and became rancid after sitting for a time on the shelf.

This limited shelf life is similar to nuts and oil. Have you ever eaten a rancid nut or smelled rancid oil? The capacity of food to become spoiled is a good thing because the foul smell and taste lets you know the value of the food is gone. However, the food industries prefer products with a longer shelf life so their products won't go bad and can be sold for a longer period of time.

Unfortunately, after the bran and germ components of the wheat berry were removed from the wheat, Americans started having diseases caused by deficiencies in B vitamins because the wheat germ, which contained the grain's nutrients, was removed from flour. Therefore, in the 1940s, vitamin enrichment of bread began.

Processed foods, like white flour, with their extended shelf life, do not go bad anymore because the natural nutrients were removed. Consequently, such foods don't benefit the human body. In fact, if we eat processed foods that do not contain nutrients, we deprive ourselves of essential vitamins and minerals. A lack of nutrients leads to malnutrition. Does it make sense to add manufactured vitamins to replace the natural nutrients stripped from the food in order to have nutritional value? God already placed the nutrients in the foods. Unfortunately, food industries take those nutrients out to extend the product's shelf life, which benefits the companies' bottom line but is detrimental to our health. No wonder our bodies are unhealthy.

Recently, a friend offered me an almond-flavored, sweet cracker. I looked at it and wondered how long ago was it created? It probably sat in a box on a shelf for months, and now it could continue to stay in my pantry indefinitely. I ate a few bites and tossed it. Afterward I experienced indigestion for several hours as my body protested the foodlike substance, which was not nourishing but damaging. Shelf life means no life.

Products made from white flour contain no nutritional value. Yet humans consume wheat products made from processed white flour all the time. Our bodies do not recognize them as food. Maybe that is why many Americans experience chronic diseases.

Sugar

Sugar-sweetened drinks raise blood-sugar levels and predispose a person to diabetes, a chronic health problem in the US. Heightened blood-sugar levels cause the release of insulin. In turn, blood-sugar levels plummet, and you feel wiped out—devoid of energy. The body releases adrenaline to counteract the low blood sugar, and this causes anxiety and even panic attacks. Could that be why the incidence of anxiety disorders has increased in our society? Blood sugar fluctuations also cause a person to be more irritable and short-tempered.

Watch the excellent documentary *The Sugar Film* about what happens to a person's body after consuming 40 grams (average sugar consumption) of sugar every day for two months. This film claims 80 percent of items in the grocery store has some form of sugar added to it.

Sugar makes our blood sugar fluctuate, and causes us to become addicted to it, which causes the harmful cycle of insulin and adrenaline release. Dr. Avena's research (in the Ted-Ed talk on sugar from step 1) revealed rats binged on sugar when it was offered. She said highly processed foods, such as refined flour, may be as problematic as sugar. Her study found that pizza, chips, and chocolate were some of the most addictive foods for the human body.[3]

Wheat and sugar comprise a large part of the American diet. At church, I sat next to a mom with a twelve-month-old baby. When she got fussy, her mother pulled out a plastic bag with toast and gave some to the child. A little later, the toothless toddler held up a graham cracker she wanted to share with me. When I left, I noticed sugar-sweetened cereal all over the floor.

All of these sugary wheat products were like crack cocaine to the child's brain, since wheat goes to the same opiate brain receptors. On a Positron Emission Tomography Scan (PET) of the human brain, the same area of the brain lit up when an obese person ingested sugar and an addict received cocaine. (To see the imaging results go to Mic.-com/articles/88015/what-happens-to-your-brain-on-sugar-explained-by-science#.huzqY8vAf.)[4] As a result, many Americans become addicted to sugar and carbohydrates, especially when we begin consuming them from a young age.

Corn Syrup

Avoid high-fructose corn syrup (HFCS), an inexpensive alternative to sugar. In the late 1970s, corn syrup was introduced into the American food system to keep manufacturing costs down and that is when obesity rates began to rise. In fact, on a graph, the increased use of HFCS mirrors the rapid increase in obesity in the US. A friend of mine who is a rheumatologist believes HFCS is a major contributor to disease in this country because after its introduction, chronic diseases began rising.

. . .

White Rice

The processing of white rice resembles wheat's story; it is processed and raises blood-sugar levels. To extend its storage life, the husk, bran, and germ are removed from the rice during the milling process, which eliminates most of the grain's nutrients. Therefore, rice is enriched just like wheat products.

Taking the beneficial nutrients out of food and enriching them is not how God intended for us to consume our vitamins and minerals. God created whole grains for our body to assimilate all the nutrients and fiber. Fiber is necessary to keep the bowels moving smoothly. It is difficult to consume the recommended daily allowance of 25–30 grams of fiber by eating processed foods such as white rice. Consuming brown and wild rice are perfectly fine because they contain the whole grain of the rice including the fiber and nutrients.

Corn

Most of the corn in the United States has been genetically modified (GMO) for resistance to insects or herbicides. Genetic engineering enables the addition of insecticidal or herbicidal proteins into the seed. Corn with herbicidal proteins allows the plant to tolerate glyphosate, which is the carcinogenic chemical in Roundup.[5]

Farmers are allowed to spray as much insecticide on GMO corn as they deem necessary. As a result, we consume corn saturated with a carcinogen. Does that sound healthy? *Do not eat corn unless it is organic!* In fact, if you see the brown spot at the tip of a cornhusk, maybe even with a little worm, that corn is not GMO and is suitable to eat. Corn that bugs like is the type of corn humans consumed for centuries.

I use to enjoy eating corn tortilla chips with salsa and guacamole. Unfortunately, the next day I always woke up with a parched mouth from excessive salt and a headache from chemicals in the corn chips. The same thing happens when I eat popcorn at a movie theater. I began thinking of corn products as loaded with a carcinogen, so I changed my mind-set and do not eat them.

. . .

Milk Products

Humans are the only mammals on earth that consume milk after the age of two. Plus, we don't even drink human milk but dairy from a cow. God made cow's milk to nurture a calf so that it can grow to be the size of a cow. Get the hint? If you stop consuming dairy products, you will naturally lose weight.

Milk, similar to wheat and rice, is denatured of its nutritional value to extend its shelf life. I remember when a milkman brought fresh milk to our front door. Food industries heat raw milk to high temperatures (pasteurization), which destroys all microorganisms and most nutrients, and they add vitamin D to it. The raw milk contained enzymes that helped with digestion. Today, lactose intolerance is high.

Consume almond, cashew, or coconut milk products instead of dairy. Don't consume soy milk or soy products unless they are organic because most of the soy crops in the United States are Roundup Ready crops. I eat coconut milk ice cream and kefir. Both are delicious, and I can't tell the difference between the cow or coconut milk products. Kefir is a fermented product that contains natural gut-friendly probiotics.

Artificial Sweeteners

Do not use artificial sweeteners. People who frequently consume sugar substitutes may be at an increased risk of excessive weight gain, type-2 diabetes, and cardiovascular disease. The sugar substitute causes a person to crave sweets. The following link is an informative *Time* magazine article about weight gain associated with the consumption of artificial sweeteners: Time.com/4859012/artificial-sweeteners-weight-loss/.[6]

One of the biggest culprits containing artificial sweeteners is diet soda. Unfortunately, many people think they are being healthy by substituting diet drinks for sugary drinks, but research indicates that artificial sweeteners in diet soda make you crave sugar and increase abdominal fat. Here is the link to a corresponding article: Medical-

Daily.com/4-dangerous-effects-artificial-sweeteners-your-health-247543.[7]

Processed Meats

The World Health Organization classified processed meats (hot dogs, ham, bacon, sausage, and some deli meats) as a group 1 carcinogen.[8] Processed meats are right up there with tobacco, asbestos, and plutonium! Most people have no idea that when they feed their child a hot dog, it is comparable to giving them a cigarette.

Different types of meat processing include salting, fermenting, curing, and smoking. Avoid purchasing any prepackaged lunch meats. Instead, bake a chicken or turkey breast and cut it up to use as lunch meat. If you buy meats at a deli, make sure the attendant cuts slices from a hunk of meat that came from an animal versus the meat being shredded and formed into a mold. For example, you could buy a natural chicken breast or thigh, but often chicken parts are processed together into a molded premade, unnatural patty, which is unhealthy.

Vegetable Oils

Most vegetable oils contain omega 6 fatty acids, which promote inflammation in the human body. Therefore, lower your consumption of omega 6 foods and increase your ingestion of omega 3 foods (which are nourishing for the brain) like avocado, nuts, and fish. Olive oil contains both omega 3 and 6 fats and is high in antioxidants, therefore, it is the preferred oil to consume.

Another beneficial oil, coconut oil, resists oxidation at high heat. Therefore, use coconut oil for high-heat cooking such as frying. Coconut oil also reduces triglycerides, LDL, and total cholesterol levels.

Processed Foods

Processed foods are the foods contained in boxes and bags in the aisles of the grocery store. These foods are far from their harvested form. *Removal of their nutrients and fiber increase their shelf life. Unfortunately, they decrease the life of the person who consumes them.* Consider them dead foods that do not benefit the body but instead harm it. *Therefore, try not to eat any processed foods out of a box or bag.* This includes cereals, chips, crackers, granola bars, cookies, etc.

However, we cannot eat perfectly all the time. We may want to eat chips or crackers with a healthy dip, or we might be a guest for dinner at someone's home. Therefore, try to eat nourishing foods at least 80 percent of the time, but the rest of the time, if you choose to eat a processed food, make sure it is organic and non-GMO.

Eat to live a healthy, bountiful life. Evaluate every single thing you eat. Is it alive or is it dead? Remember, shelf life means no life.

Peanuts

Contrary to popular belief, peanuts are not a nut but a type of a vegetable called a legume (i.e., pea or bean). They grow in the ground and don't come from a tree. I also do not recommend consuming peanut butter because it is hard to digest and many people are allergic to it.

There is a peanut field right behind my house. The peanuts are dug up and left on the ground to dry for a couple of weeks. During that time, they get soaked from rain, and I can only imagine how much mold may grow on them in the humid Florida weather. Almond or cashew nuts and butter are better choices.

Two weeks after my sister got off sugar and refined carbohydrates, she ate some peanuts. Afterward she experienced a stomachache. She had eaten peanuts all her life and never noticed the harmful effects. After she weaned herself off sugar and wheat, she was more aware of the effects different foods had on her body. With time you will become more aware of this as well.

Margarine

Margarine most likely contains trans-fat, which increases the risk of heart disease, and free radicals, which contribute to numerous health problems including cancer. Instead use organic butter, olive oil, and coconut oil.

Canned Goods

Bisphenol (BPA) is an industrial chemical used to make some plastics. Canned foods are lined with BPA to prevent erosion of the can. An ongoing debate ensues between scientific studies and the Federal Drug Administration (FDA) regarding whether the level of BPA found in canned foods is safe for humans. Nonetheless, when we eat canned foods, we are exposed to this chemical. In fact, scientific studies found BPA in the urine of study participants who consumed canned food within the past twenty-four hours.[10] The FDA banned the use of certain BPA-based materials used in infant bottles, sippy cups, and infant formula packaging.[11] Therefore, try not to eat canned goods. Instead, purchase fresh vegetables, fruits, and dried beans. Foods preserved in glass (such as spaghetti sauce), not cans, is a better option.

Microwavable Foods

Many food products are microwaveable—from popcorn to frozen dinners. However, when you microwave your food or beverages the microwave alters the food, decreases hemoglobin, and raises bad cholesterol. Read further evidence in this article: Mercola.com/article/microwave/hazards2.htm.[12] Therefore, I recommend reheating leftovers in a toaster oven and limiting your use of the microwave. It takes three minutes to warm up leftovers in a toaster oven.

For popcorn, simple cook organic, non-GMO kernels in a stovetop pan with a lid. Add a little olive or coconut oil and in three minutes the kernels pop. This is about the same amount of time it takes to pop microwave popcorn. I top my popcorn with half organic butter and half olive oil, along with kelp and dulse seaweed sprinkles and sea salt.

CLEAN OUT THE PANTRY

Step 3 includes cleaning out the pantry and refrigerator. The most enlightening resource for this cleanout is a fifteen-minute video by Dr. Daniel Amen who coauthored *The Daniel Plan*. Watch "What's in Your Pantry" on YouTube.com.[13]

Remove the following unhealthy items from your pantry:

- Wheat—anything that contains wheat
- Sugar-sweetened drinks—like soda, fruit juice, Gatorade (Flavored waters with no calories are okay to keep and finish, but after they are gone it is best to drink water. If you need to, add a slice of lemon and stevia to your water.)
- Sugar—white sugar, high-fructose corn syrup—remove any item with greater than 10 grams of sugar per serving. Unfortunately, sugar does not have a recommended daily allowance.
- Rice—white rice (brown and wild rice are fine)
- Corn—all non-organic corn products such as tortilla chips and popcorn (Organic corn products are fine to consume.)
- Artificial sweeteners—saccharin, aspartame or Equal/NutraSweet, sucralose or Splenda (It is okay to keep honey, maple syrup, agave, stevia, xylitol, coconut sugar, monk fruit sugar.)
- Oils—eliminate all oils except olive oil (use when cooking at low temperatures) and coconut oil (use when cooking at high temperatures)
- Any processed food in a box or bag such as chips, crackers, cookies, and cereal unless it is organic and you choose to make this an exception

- Foods that contain partially hydrogenated vegetable oil, high-fructose corn syrup, or monosodium glutamate (MSG). Food labels disguise MSG through the following names: flavors; flavoring; enzymes; hydrolyzed, autolyzed yeast; barley malt; hydrolyzed vegetable protein; maltodextrin; natural seasonings; and glutamate.

CLEAN OUT THE REFRIGERATOR

Let's move on to cleaning out the refrigerator. Remove the following unhealthy items from your refrigerator.

- Wheat products
- Processed meats such as ham, bacon, sausage, hot dogs, and lunch meat
- Soft drinks and fruit juices—they are loaded with sugar
- Check the ingredients of condiments. If one contains high-fructose corn syrup, throw it out. Health-food stores carry better condiment substitutes, such as organic mayonnaise.
- Margarine—organic butter is a healthier choice
- All milk products except plain Greek yogurt, which contains probiotics

CLEAN OUR YOUR FREEZER

Let's open up that freezer and see what is inside. Throw out the following unhealthy products:

- Wheat products
- Dairy products (Replace your dairy products, such as ice cream, with coconut, almond, or cashew milk items.)
- Packaged frozen meals (while convenient, even the "healthy" brands of frozen foods are processed)

CLEAN OUT YOUR EMOTIONS

Food and emotions are intrinsically tied together for most of us, so we need to do an emotional check when we begin to clean out the foods that have previously brought us comfort.

Interestingly, original sin began with eating. It was probably a sweet fruit, like a fig. In Genesis 3:4–7 we read, "'You will not certainly die,' the serpent said to the woman. 'For God knows that when you eat from it your eyes will be opened, and you will be like God, knowing good and evil.' When the woman saw that the fruit of the tree was good for food and pleasing to the eye, and also desirable for gaining wisdom, she took some and ate it. She also gave some to her husband, who was with her, and he ate it. Then the eyes of both of them were opened, and they realized they were naked; so they sewed fig leaves together and made coverings for themselves" (NIV).

God gave us food to nourish our bodies. Yet food can be used for the wrong reasons. We may eat because we are sad, bored, stressed out, depressed, or happy. As we engage in emotional eating, we turn to food, instead of to God, to appease ourselves. If we feel abandoned, food can be our friend. We can swallow our angry feelings with food, instead of feeling the emotions we don't want to deal with. Food can provide an emotional escape from negative feelings.

To help you go more in-depth into the root cause of a dysfunctional relationship with food, I wrote *Christian Study Guide for 7 Steps to Get Off Sugar and Carbohydrates*. It goes into the issues of childhood wounds, abuse, and generational bondage. Getting to the root cause is vital to resolving the food issue once and for all.

In your journal (appendix 3 or *Healthy Living Journal*) document why you eat. Is it because of hunger or to relieve stress? Do you have a deep emotional wound that needs healing? If you do, journal and talk to God about it. Is there someone you need to forgive? Maybe you have a big hole in your heart that you are filling with food. God is our ultimate healer, take your wounds to him and ask him to heal you. Forgive as Jesus instructed us to do.

Sometimes we engage in mindless eating, where we munch on

something without being hungry. When a person is bored, she may look in the refrigerator or pantry but can't find anything appealing. If this happens to you, food is not what you need. First, drink two glasses of water, as you may be thirsty and don't realize it. Next, your soul may be longing for a connection with God, so spend time with him. Journal your thoughts.

Are you eating because of a negative emotion you do not want to deal with? Don't escape from negative feelings through undesirable eating. Instead, recognize dysfunctional eating behaviors and confront tough issues in your life. Bring those problems to God and be honest with him about what you experience. Each time you recognize emotional eating, clean out your emotions with God. Then you can disengage the connection between eating and feelings.

Your value to God is not determined by what you weigh. Your body is the temple of the Holy Spirit. Do not try to overcome inappropriate eating on your own, instead call on the power of the Holy Spirit to empower you to change. With God's help, you can overcome and succeed. Opening up to your accountability partner and support group is also instrumental in attaining success over emotional eating, as they can remind you of God's power in your life and can pray with you to reconnect with God when you are fighting the spiritual battle around food and emotions.

Stress also causes us to turn to food. We live in a fast-paced world where we eat on the run. We no longer have traditional meals prepared from scratch at home. Unfortunately, food industries are cooking our food for us today.

Determine the stressors (things that cause you stress) in your life, and list them in your journal. Can you do something about the stressors? Evaluate each one and brainstorm on how to minimize them. Pray to God and ask him to enlighten you and help you. Ask your accountability partner or support group for help and prayer in dealing with your stressors

How do you cope with stress? Do you tend to deal with it through undesirable eating habits? If so, recognize this and choose to do something about your stress level. Can you eliminate a stressor in your life? Some stress-relieving activities include praying with your prayer partner, enjoying a massage, journaling, and calling a friend.

Do you exercise? Exercising, a positive coping strategy for dealing with stress, burns off adrenaline and improves sleep. Do you engage in relaxation techniques such as Christian yoga or meditation? Yoga and meditation calm the mind and body. I created several Christian yoga products including DVDs, books, and card decks available at: ChristianYoga.com.

Stress tends to make people crave carbohydrates, sugary comfort foods, and junk food. These types of processed foods give you a sugar rush, but then your blood sugar crashes, and you feel rotten. The feelings from the blood-sugar fluctuation cause even more anxiety.

Plan Ahead to Avoid Emotional and Stress Eating

To develop an effective plan, document in your journal what you eat and why. A list of items to record in your journal is provided in appendix 3. Record any negative emotions you experience and determine if you eat because of your feelings. Connect the dots between your eating habits and emotions. If you discover you are engaging in emotional eating, you need to substitute it with another behavior. Also record in your journal the stressors in your life and when you are feeling stressed, so you can replace unhealthy food choices with positive behaviors.

When you recognize you are about to emotionally eat or eat out of stress, set the timer for ten minutes and spend that time with God. Express your emotions and ask him to transform your mind. Recite Bible verses out loud. After the timer rings, if you still want to eat, go on a walk, call your accountability partner, or put in a Christian yoga DVD. Break the cycle of the emotions you feel and your conditioned response to eating. A list of Food Addiction Battle Strategies is provided in appendix 10.

TAKING STEP 3: CLEAN OUT

Now that you've made it to step 3, you should feel more confident about incorporating new food choices into your healthier lifestyle. Make sure you take the following action steps:

1. Schedule a date to clean out your pantry, refrigerator, and freezer.

Date to clean out:Date accomplished:

Pantry _____

Refrigerator _____

Freezer _____

2. Cleaning out your emotions entails several steps. Do you have your journal yet? You can purchase the *Healthy Living Journal* at Susan-UNeal.com/Shop. Are you journaling what you eat and determining why you are eating? Please see the list of items you should be recording in appendix 3. Be sure to journal your thoughts and emotions too.

3. List the things in your life which cause you stress.

_____

_____

4. Think about ways that you can reduce or eliminate these stressors. List those ideas:

_____

_____

5. List some activities you would like to do to decrease your stress:

. . .

----

7 Steps to Get Off Sugar and Carbohydrates:

Step 1. Decide to improve your health through proper nutrition.-substitute positive behaviors for

Step 2. Acquire a support system and knowledge to help make a lifestyle change.

Step 3. Clean out your pantry and refrigerator by removing unhealthy foods and clean out your emotions.

STEP 4: PURCHASE HEALTHY FOODS AND AN ANTI-CANDIDA CLEANSE

Decide—>Acquire—>Clean Out—>**Purchase**—>Plan—>Prepare—>Improve

You decided (step 1) to make a lifestyle change and improve your health. Acquiring knowledge (step 2) about changing your eating habits and identifying your support system takes time but will help you keep your commitment to this decision. Cleaning out (step 3) the pantry and refrigerator was a chore, but not as difficult as cleaning out your emotions. Now it is time to *purchase* (step 4) groceries based on the healthy eating guidelines specified in this chapter.

When I told my sister that a low-glycemic diet meant she could no longer eat wheat, rice, or anything with sugar, she asked, "What *can* I eat?"

I told her, "You can eat vegetables, beans, meat, nuts, seeds, and low-sugar fruit."

To her (and probably you), this was a total change in her diet, since she ate primarily high glycemic foods. This change in eating habits felt radical and seemed limiting to her, but God gave us an incredible variety of food to enjoy and sustain our bodies, including a vast selection of different vegetables and fruits.

HEALTHY FOODS TO PURCHASE

In step 2 we reviewed a long list of resources so you can continue to educate yourself about making this lifestyle change. However, I believe our most significant resource is the Bible, so let's check out what God told us to eat. "Then God said, 'Look! I have given you every seed-bearing plant throughout the earth and all the fruit trees for your food'" (Genesis 1:29). We know what a fruit tree is, but what exactly is a seed-bearing plant? It produces seeds that can be planted again, such as grains and vegetables.

Fruits are so sweet and delicious they can be called God's candy. Instead of eating a dish of ice cream, eat a juicy strawberry, tangy green apple, or crunchy pomegranate. Fruits are not just juicy and sweet but also provide the body with the fiber, vitamins, and minerals our bodies need to be healthy. God is an artist who created different sizes, shapes, and vibrant colors of fruit.

God also created over a hundred different vegetables because the human body needs various types of nutrients essential for proper growth and performance. For example, spinach contains vitamins A and K, whereas broccoli is full of vitamin E. God gave us a variety to choose from to ensure we get the proper amounts of fiber, vitamins, and minerals.

Grains provide carbohydrates the body uses for fuel or energy. Similar to gas in a car. God offered us an assortment of grains to choose from: amaranth, barley, buckwheat, millet, oats, quinoa, rice, rye, wheat, and wild rice. Two grains I do not recommend are white rice and wheat, because of the way they are processed today, with the nutrients stripped away; all others are beneficial.

Nuts are excellent sources of protein, similar to meat. Again, God created numerous varieties to choose from including almond, brazil, cashew, chestnut, hazelnut, macadamia, pecan, pistachio, pine, and walnut. Be sure to buy raw nuts because they contain more nutrition in their natural, raw form, not roasted, salted, or sugar coated. Instead, taste the natural flavor of almonds, pecans, and walnuts. God gave us nuts to eat, and they are full of omega 3 oils, which are essential for brain function.

As previously explained, peanuts are not a nut but a type of vegetable called a legume (i.e., pea or bean). They grow in the ground and don't come from a tree. I do not recommend consuming products made with peanuts because it is hard to digest and many people are allergic to it. Other legumes (beans, lentils, and peas) may be difficult for some people to digest, but generally don't cause allergic reactions.

God gave us chia, flax, hemp, poppy, pumpkin, sesame, and sunflower seeds. Seeds are full of trace minerals the human body needs but in small amounts. Since God made us, he knows what our bodies require, and he provides it for us in different ways.

Fruits and vegetables are seasonal, which means each season (spring, summer, fall, winter) different crops are harvested. In the south, strawberries ripen in early spring. Okra and peas grow best in the summer. Pumpkins mature in the fall. Citrus fruit is picked in the winter when our bodies require more vitamin C to prevent colds. God supplies a selection of fruit and vegetables each season, and we should eat the ones that ripen in that season. Not only will we get the nutrients we need for that season but we won't tire of eating the same type of food all year long.

Sometimes we get into the habit of eating the same sort of food over and over again, but it is healthier to eat an assortment to get a variety of nutrients. We can choose from a vast number of fruits, vegetables, grains, nuts, and seeds, and each is unique in its flavor and amount of nutrients. God knew what he was doing when he created these nutrient-rich foods for us to consume. They not only provide what our body needs but they are delicious to enjoy as well. God wants us to enjoy all of his creation.

Yet God never put food in a box or bag and had them sit on the shelf for months. He didn't label them with an expiration date. He gave humans a vast selection of food since their bodies need a broad range of nutrients to function correctly. *By eating different foods from each food category (vegetable, fruit, grain, nut, seed), you take proper care of your body.* God did not give us vitamin pills either. Instead he created fresh food right from the plant or tree and loaded them with vitamins and minerals so our bodies will function at their highest potential.

After the flood, God introduced meat into the human diet. As God directed Noah in Genesis 9:2–3, "'All wild animals and birds and fish will be afraid of you,' God told him; 'for I have placed them in your power, and they are yours to use for food, in addition to grain and vegetables'" (TLB). After humans began consuming meat, their life-span significantly shortened. I am not saying we shouldn't eat meat. However, there are healthy protein alternatives to meat such as nuts and beans.

When you purchase meat, make sure it is organic, grass fed, or free range with no hormones or antibiotics. I think the antibiotics we consume from our meat also harm our gut flora.

We do not need to consume meat at every meal. From a blood analysis, my sister discovered she had an excess amount of protein. Too much protein in a person's diet causes the body to extract calcium from the bones and send it into the bloodstream to balance its pH.[1] This calcium leaching weakens a person's bones and is a factor in osteoporosis. In fact, incidences of osteoporosis in third-world countries with a low-protein diet are lower than industrialized nations.[2]

One summer I bought a new fruit and vegetable every week at the grocery store. It was an excellent experience for our children and me as I got out of the rut of cooking the same meals over and over, and we found different foods we liked such as red cabbage, star fruit, and bok choy.

HEALTHY EATING GUIDELINES

The following healthy eating guidelines are my secret to maintaining optimal weight and brain health. This is a low-carbohydrate, low-glycemic, anti-inflammatory eating plan, which is the type of diet recommended for improving memory and cognition and preventing and reversing type-2 diabetes. A summary of Healthy Eating Guidelines is included in appendix 5.

A low-glycemic diet does not raise blood sugar or insulin levels. Foods high in carbohydrates cause a release of glucose into the bloodstream and a corresponding rise in insulin. Avoid the following high-carbohydrate foods: cakes, crackers, sugary cereals and drinks, flours, bread products, jellies/jams, and refined potato products. These types of foods are addictive.

Low-carbohydrate, anti-inflammatory dietary guidelines include:

- About 50 percent of food items are fresh organic vegetables.
- Eat one fresh, raw serving of low-glycemic fruit per day. Low-glycemic fruits include green apples, berries, cherries, pears, plums, and grapefruit.
- Do not always eat cooked foods. Eat a couple of servings of raw vegetables every day. Have a salad for lunch with either nuts or meat. When eating out, order a salad or coleslaw as sides, since both are raw.
- Another 25 percent of your daily food intake should come from an animal or vegetable protein such as beans, nuts, and lean meats. Fish is exceptionally nutritious. Try to eat it once a week.
- A variety of different nuts and seeds are excellent sources of protein, minerals, and essential fatty acids.
- Avoid sugar, flour, rice, pasta, and bread. Instead, eat more fruits, vegetables, and low-glycemic grains such as quinoa and pearled barley.
- Do not eat sugary cereals. Instead, eat oatmeal, fruit, or

granola. Be careful, as the sugar content of granola may be high. My favorite granola recipe appears in appendix 4.

- Try not to eat anything containing more than 10 grams of sugar in one serving.
- Eat nontraditional grains such as quinoa, amaranth, pearled barley, wild rice, and organic oats.
- Eat cultured foods such as kimchi, sauerkraut, and cultured plain Greek yogurt since they contain natural probiotics. Add one to two tablespoons of these foods to a meal twice a week or eat the yogurt as a snack. Personally, I take a probiotic capsule every day.
- Replace undesirable ingredients with whole foods. *The Daniel Plan Cookbook* by Rick Warren provides a chart titled Foods and Ingredients to Avoid and suggests replacements.[3] A few recommendations from this book include:
- Replace sugary snacks with nuts, nut butter, dark chocolate, and plain Greek yogurt with berries.
- Replace condiments and sauces containing MSG or high-fructose corn syrup with spices, vinegar, and herbs.
- Replace table salt with kosher or sea salt.
- Replace fried foods with baked foods.

My additional healthy eating tips include:

- Make homemade granola from organic oats (recipe in appendix 4). For breakfast, I add fresh berries to a bowl of granola.
- Buy or whip up a flavorful dip like hummus or guacamole to eat with a platter of fresh vegetables (not chips or pita bread).
- Substitute beans for meat for some meals.
- Squeeze a slice of lemon and add a couple drops of liquid stevia into a glass of water. It is like drinking lemonade.
- Boil eggs and keep them in the refrigerator for a snack.

- Chew your food thoroughly because this is where digestion begins.

Please try not to be overwhelmed by all of this information. Guide your eating with the 80/20 percent rule. *If you eat healthy 80 percent of the time and not so healthy 20 percent of the time, this will probably be an improvement.*

I don't eat perfectly, but I try. With God's help, I attempt not to eat more than 10 grams of sugar at one sitting. If I mess up, the next day I get to start new, as indicated in Lamentations 3:22–23, "Because of the LORD's great love we are not consumed, for his compassions never fail. They are new every morning; great is your faithfulness" (NIV).

Each morning as I wake up, my body tells me how well I ate the previous day. If I did not experience any blood sugar fluctuations, I have a clear mind and abundant energy. The incredible sensation of how God created our bodies to feel motivates me to continue to eat well every day. I am more productive when I eat healthy foods.

While shopping at a grocery store, shop along the edges of the store in the dairy, meat, and produce sections. Stay away from the center of the store where processed foods experience an extended shelf life. Remember, *a long shelf life means the nutritional value of the food has been removed.* Otherwise, the food becomes rancid at some point. If a food spoils, it is beneficial, but if it does not spoil, it contains no nutrients.

HEALTHY SUBSTITUTIONS TO PURCHASE

Many unhealthy food choices can be replaced with healthy alternatives that are whole, unprocessed, and natural. In addition to the replacements mentioned above from Rick Warren's book *The Daniel Plan Cookbook*, the following sections offer a number of options to replace the unhealthy foods you eliminated in step 3 with healthy, flavorful foods as God intended.

. . .

Sugar Substitutes

Substitute sugar with a natural sweetener, stevia, which is an herb. Purchase stevia in a health food store because popular stevia products at the grocery store are too refined. Another option is local honey. However, honey raises blood sugar levels. I use a powder form of stevia for baking. Also, I found a natural sweetener with zero calories that rates zero on the glycemic index—Lakanto Monkfruit Sweetener (Lakanto.com/); which is made from monk fruit.

In the following list I rank the best natural sugar substitutes based on their glycemic index:

stevia-0

monk fruit sweetener-0

xylitol-12

agave-15

coconut sugar-35

honey-50

maple syrup-54

Try out these different sweeteners. Choose a natural, low-glycemic sweetener that you can live with and use it sparingly.

Pasta Substitutes

My sister wanted to know what she would use for pasta in her new lifestyle. I told her to buy spaghetti squash, use shirataki noodles, or spiralize zucchini. Spaghetti squash can sit on a counter for a couple of weeks, just like a box of spaghetti, and it is simple to cook. Cut it in half, scrape the seeds out of the center, and put it, cut side up, on a baking sheet with 1/4 inch of water in the pan. Bake at 350° for 30–40 minutes. When done, scrape the inside with a fork for a low-glycemic "spaghetti." The squash absorbs any flavor you put on it, such as shrimp scampi or spaghetti sauce. This vegetable also tastes great as a side dish with olive oil and seasonings.

To spiralize zucchini, purchase a spiralizer. Push the zucchini through the device and out comes your zucchini noodles. For shirataki noodles, cook them as directed on the package and add your sauce. Again, zucchini and shirataki noodles absorb the flavor of the sauce added to them.

Meat Substitutes

Fish, nuts, and beans are excellent sources of protein, which are healthier for you than meat. Every week, prepare a few meals with one of these meat substitutes as the primary protein source. Serve fish one night, beans another, and nuts on your salad for a third.

Nuts also contain omega-3 fatty acids. Pecans grow in the south, walnuts in the Carolinas, macadamia nuts in Hawaii. What types of nuts grow in your area? I recommend that during the nut-harvesting season in your area you purchase a lot of nuts. Every year, I freeze at least twelve pint jars of pecans. I use one every month. This is an excellent way to obtain local, fresh nuts at an economical price.

Beans are another great substitute for meat. I recommend cooking one meal a week with beans as the main source of protein. Appendix 4 contains a lot of flavorful recipes that include beans. Dried beans are better for you than canned. Soak beans overnight and throw out the water. The water contains the beans' gas-causing substance. If you need to, take a digestive enzyme from the health food store to prevent flatulence.

Try to substitute fish for meat. Fresh wild-caught salmon is available in upper-end grocery stores from July–October. I try to serve this twice a month during this time. Plan on preparing fish once a week. Leftover fish is not as palatable as fresh, so I included a delicious fish stew recipe in appendix 4.

Another alternative to meat is whole grain quinoa, which contains five grams of protein in one serving (1/2 cup cooked). I sauté fresh vegetables and combine them with quinoa for a satisfying meal that takes only twenty minutes to prepare. Countless vegetable combinations can be created: sautéed scallions, mushrooms, and spinach along with sunflower and pumpkin seeds; sautéed onion, bell peppers, and kale with a fresh avocado on top; sautéed bok choy, snow peas, and carrots with cashews and sesame seeds.

Dairy Substitutes

It is best not to consume milk products. However, several healthy dairy substitutes include almond, cashew, and coconut milk. Personally, I enjoy the flavor of toasted coconut almond blend, which combines both of these milks. If you like soy milk, be sure to purchase organic soy products as soy is one of the Roundup Ready crops I discussed in step 2.

WATER

Most people do not nourish and cleanse their bodies with an adequate amount of water on a daily basis. The human body is comprised of 75 percent water, and we can't survive for more than a few days without it. Some people think drinking tea, juice, soda, or other drinks will hydrate their body, but they don't. In fact, caffeinated beverages are a diuretic, which causes you to urinate more frequently and lose fluid. Drink an average of eight glasses of water per day.

However, your water requirements depend upon your size. Various sources recommend: "Drink half your weight in ounces every day." Using this formula, a 130-pound person should drink eight glasses of water. (130/2 = 65 ounces; 65/8 ounces (1 cup) = 8 glasses.)

Scheduling when to drink water throughout the day can be tricky because it is best to drink on an empty stomach. Therefore, drink two glasses of water early in the morning before breakfast. Drink two more glasses before lunch. In the afternoon, when you desire an afternoon snack, drink two glasses of water, which will help curb your appetite. Consume your last two glasses before dinner. Yes, you will go to the bathroom more often; don't think of it as a burden but as a process whereby toxins expel from your body. Don't drink any beverage after dinner to prevent getting up during the night to go to the bathroom.

If you do not consume an adequate amount of water, your body suffers the consequences. Some common symptoms of dehydration include constipation, fatigue, dry skin and mouth, bladder and kidney problems, and high blood pressure since the blood is thicker. Our blood is 90 percent water.

My mother and aunt did not like water. They preferred sweet tea and coffee. My aunt contracted bladder cancer and my mother experienced frequent urinary tract infections (UTI). Water helps cleanse the body of toxins. If we don't drink enough water to flush the toxins out of our kidneys and bladder, the toxins accumulate in these organs and cause infection and disease.

Consider these additional tips for your water intake each day:

- Do not drink with meals because the fluid dilutes digestive enzymes, which secrete to break down the food. Instead, drink between meals, usually three hours after a meal, which gives time for food digestion. You may drink up to ten minutes before you eat.
- Drink an average of eight glasses of water every day or the recommended amount for your weight. Other than coffee or tea, water should be the only beverage consumed. Do not count coffee and tea toward the number of glasses of water.
- If you feel hungry, drink water. Scientists reported that two 8-ounce glasses of water is an effective weight loss strategy because many times when a person feels hungry, they are actually thirsty.[4] So drink water and see if that fills you up before eating. You may be pleasantly surprised.

The *Healthy Living Journal* contains a Water Tracker Chart for you to keep track of how much water your drink on a daily basis.

FOODS THAT CAUSE INFLAMMATION

Some medical literature claims inflammation is the root of chronic disease. Where do you think inflammation comes from? It generates from what we put into our bodies and most likely from the food we ingest.

We eat many foods that are far from the product that they were when it was harvested. The human body does not recognize some of these so-called foods as beneficial and so it reacts negatively and causes inflammation. Inflammation causes a wide-range of negative effects across many systems in the body. It is important to identify what food is causing a negative effect in you. A week after my sister stopped eating wheat, her joint pain went away. This is an example of the positive effects that occur when you eliminate inflammatory foods.

Limit milk products because they cause mucus formation and inflammation. In fact, dairy is recognized as one of the top five inflammatory foods.[5] If you are lactose intolerant, like me, do not eat or drink milk products. However, if you choose to ingest dairy, take a lactaid tablet to help with digestion.

Sugar and wheat are two other major inflammation-causing foods. I taught The Daniel Plan by Rick Warren, which recommends you stop eating sugar, wheat, and milk products for one week. Then you reintroduce one of those foods at a time to determine any adverse effects. Every time I reintroduced dairy products, I experienced additional phlegm and postnasal drip. I realized milk products caused inflammation in my system, yet I had consumed them for fifty years. It is vital for you to figure out what may be causing an inflammatory response in your body too. When you track the foods you eat and your bodies response to them you determine which foods cause inflammation in your body.

Our food today contains all sorts of chemicals and additives. Conversely, a vegetable or piece of fruit does not contain artificial additives except for the pesticides and herbicides sprayed on them. I do not want to consume any glyphosate (carcinogen) residue contained in Roundup Ready crops such as oats, wheat, soy, corn, or sugar beets. Consequently, I buy organic and I recommend you do too.

If you choose to purchase nonorganic fruits and vegetables, understand that the thinner the skin, the deeper the pesticide and herbicide penetrate the fruit. For example, strawberries soak up the chemicals, but bananas have a thicker skin and therefore do not.

I met a woman at a conference who suffered from inflammation so severely she experienced swelling throughout her whole body, including her fingers. As we reviewed the three primary food culprits —sugar, wheat, and dairy—she told me it couldn't be dairy because she loved cheese and ate it her whole life. I explained to her that a high consumption of cheese might be causing an inflammatory response in her body, but she wouldn't find out until she stopped eating it for at least a week and observed her symptoms when she reintroduced it.

If you think there may be a specific food causing you problematic symptoms in your body, eliminate it for at least a week. When you reintroduce it, be sure to record in your journal what symptoms you experience. If you would like me to coach you during this process, I offer healthy and wellness coaching services at SusanUNeal.com/Health-Coaching.

GUT HEALTH

You may have an imbalance in the flora of your gut if you crave sugar, alcohol, wheat, and processed foods. If your gut is not healthy, you are not healthy. An excellent resource that will explain what occurs when you develop an intestinal imbalance is *The Body Ecology Diet* by Donna Gates.[6] Check out her website Bodyecology.com.

After taking antibiotics and steroids due to an abscessed tooth, I suffered from candidiasis (an overgrowth of yeast) in my gut. A person's abdomen becomes distended when they have an overgrowth of yeast. Is your stomach distended? Candidiasis is like a parasite growing inside of you, and you don't even know it. The Candida begins to grow roots into the lining of your GI tract and makes you crave carbs because that is what it eats. Stopping this parasite's cravings and killing the Candida is tough, but I did and you can too!

To kill the overgrowth of yeast, I stopped eating specific foods for eight months. These foods included: sugar, fruit, wheat, and rice. I had to limit my alcohol consumption to vodka because it is distilled not fermented, therefore, it does not contain a grain like wheat. Most, if not all, alcoholics have candidiasis.

I was successful in killing the yeast in my colon, but I still cannot eat foods with high sugar content or the Candida starts to grow again. I can tell it is growing when I start to crave carbohydrates and feel tired.

During the eight months of my strict anti-Candida diet, I also took large doses of probiotics (up to 100 billion units/day). Probiotics for colon and vaginal health helped target those problem areas. Today, I still take probiotics but not such a large dose. The *Grain Brain* author, Dr. David Perlmutter, recommends taking a probiotic that contains at least ten billion active cultures from at least ten different strains including Lactobacillus acidophilus and Bifidobacteruim.[7] Therefore, I change the brand of my probiotic every time I purchase a new one, so I can get a wide-range of beneficial microorganisms.

To determine if you have a candida overgrowth in your gut, take the Candida Quiz at CandiQuiz.com.

FIBER

Be sure you get enough fiber. Most of us do not consume the recommended 25–30 grams of fiber per day. You should have a bowel movement (BM) at least once a day. Meat slows digestion. As you increase the fruits and vegetables in your diet, having a daily BM will not be a problem.

We need something like a broom to sweep out the inside of our colons and remove the buildup of fecal matter. Our natural broom is raw fruits and vegetables. Every spring when my garden produces its first crop, my number of BMs increase as fresh vegetables sweep my colon. Eating fresh fruits and vegetables is a natural method to cleanse a colon. You may notice an increase in your BMs as you increase your consumption of vegetables instead of processed foods. If you experience constipation, supplement with oxygenated magnesium, ground flaxseed, or other natural fiber supplements from a health food store.

WEEKLY MENU PLANNING

Planning my weekly menu takes about an hour, and I usually do this on Sunday afternoons. If the weather is nice, I sit by the pool and get my vitamin D naturally from the sun. Twenty minutes of sun without sunscreen is beneficial and won't cause sun damage. I use one recipe book and something to write on, or I use the notes app on my smartphone.

Create two lists—a grocery list and a menu for the breakfast, lunch, snack, and dinner for the week. Post the menu on the refrigerator. Next, hit the grocery store or local farmer's market. Your family will appreciate your planning and food preparation, and being prepared will keep you from making unhealthy impulsive choices when you grocery shop.

Be sure to purchase an anti-Candida cleanse from a health food store or online. An attendant at the health food store can tell you the best cleanse that they carry. Food addiction and Candida overgrowth are the most likely reasons a person craves sugary foods and refined carbohydrates.

JOURNAL

During each step of this lifestyle change, continue to journal. Have you purchased the *Healthy Living Journal* or created your own journal yet? The journal's purpose is to record what you eat, drink, and exercise, as well as the emotional and spiritual implications you have with food. See appendix 3 for specific documentation suggestions.

Keep track in your journal of the number of glasses of water you consume per day. Also write down how frequently you exercise a week. This tracking is important for your physical health, yet one of the most valuable components of your journal is what takes place in your mind. When you choose to binge, what have you told yourself? Write it down. Just as it is important to determine the nutritional content of food, it is vital to figure out the strongholds you have in your mind. Understanding yourself and what your inner voice tells you about food is instrumental to determine the root cause of dysfunctional food habits.

Jesus told us in John 10:10, "The thief's purpose is to steal, kill and destroy. My purpose is to give life in all its fullness" (TLB). Are you living life to its fullness? Is your health or weight impeding you from embracing a healthy, bountiful life? Remember to evaluate every single thing you purchase to eat. Is it dead or is it alive?

TAKING STEP 4: PURCHASE

This step helps you purchase the right foods and plan for buying and eating the right foods to continue on this healthy journey. Make sure you take the following action steps:

1. Become familiar with the healthy eating guidelines provided in step 4 and appendix 5. Print out a printable version of this appendix at SusanUNeal.com/appendix.
2. Determine what alternatives you will use for sugar, pasta, dairy, and to some extend meat.
3. Plan your menu for the week and a corresponding grocery list.
4. Purchase healthy, organic fruits, vegetables, whole grains, nuts, seeds, fish, and meats.
5. Take the Candida Quiz at CandiQuiz.com.
6. Buy and implement an anti-Candida cleanse.
7. If you haven't done so already, purchase the *Healthy Living Journal* or create your own journal.

7 Steps to Get Off Sugar and Carbohydrates:

Step 1. Decide to improve your health through proper nutrition.

Step 2. Acquire a support system and knowledge to help make a lifestyle change.

Step 3. Clean out your pantry and refrigerator by removing unhealthy foods and clean out your emotions.

Step 4. Purchase healthy foods and an anti-Candida cleanse.

5

STEP 5: PLAN FOR THE START DATE

Decide—>Acquire—>Clean Out—>Purchase—>**Plan**—>Prepare—>Improve

We need both a physical and spiritual *plan* for getting off sugar and carbohydrates. We are complex beings with a body, mind, spirit, and soul. From step 2, we understand the biochemical component of addiction to wheat and sugar. However, the spiritual component remains—that these products may be a stronghold we turn to instead of God to meet our needs. A seven-day plan of how to wean our physical bodies off of these highly addictive products and a detailed five-step spiritual plan for resisting temptation is examined in step 5.

Once you have eliminated unhealthy foods (step 3) and purchased good, nutritious foods (step 4), begin changing your eating habits by following the seven-day outline below. If you work, I recommend starting this program on a Wednesday so you can rest on the weekend. The first few days will be difficult (similar to a drug addict coming off of a drug), but with the help of Christ, prayer, an accountability partner, and these guidelines you can succeed! I included scripture verses in appendix 1 for you to recite when tempted to eat unhealthy foods.

My sister followed the Seven-Day Eating Plan. She started the plan on a Wednesday. She experienced a headache on Saturday and Monday after eliminating sugar and processed foods. Fortunately, by Monday evening her bothersome symptoms associated with stopping the sugar addiction subsided. After a week of being off sugar, she felt more energetic. She also noticed her joint pain was gone and she no longer passed gas. The first week was tough, but she did it.

You can succeed too—my sister did, I did—so let's ask God to help you: "Dear heavenly Father, please be with the reader who wants to change the way she eats so she can live the abundant life you planned for her. Please give her the power and strength to succeed. For Psalm 138:3 states, 'As soon as I pray, you answer me; you encourage me by giving me strength.' Please Lord, give her strength. Through Jesus's holy name we pray. Amen."

Appendix 6 includes a summary of this Seven-Day Eating Plan.

SEVEN-DAY EATING PLAN

Day 1 (Start on Wednesday)

1. Consume Water

Drink up to two cups of coffee or tea per day, but no more. The only other beverage you should drink is filtered water. I use a filter on my refrigerator water dispenser and a water filter on a pitcher. Before breakfast drink two glasses of water, two before lunch, two midafternoon, and two more before dinner. Do not drink during meals and do not drink anything after dinner. Drink up to ten minutes before eating.

2. Take a Probiotic

Begin taking a probiotic every day. I usually buy several probiotics from a health food store with at least ten different strains of beneficial bacteria, and I take a different one each day to vary the flora in my gastrointestinal system. I store my probiotics in the refrigerator door. After I take a probiotic, I move the bottle to a different shelf, so I can keep track of the one I took last.

3. Stop Eating High-Sugar Foods

Stop eating anything containing greater than 10 grams of sugar per serving. The American Heart Association recommends you limit your calories from sugar to no more than half of your total calories, which is a lot. For most women in the US that should be no more than 24 grams of sugar or 100 calories per day. For men it is 36 grams of sugar or 150 calories from sugar per day. Check labels for the number of grams of sugar per serving size.

Day 2

1. Eliminate Wheat

Do not eat anything containing wheat. No more bagels, toast, pancakes, biscuits, pasta, pretzels, crackers, cookies, cake, or pie. Eliminating wheat is like going off a drug. Be aware that you may experience the following symptoms for a few days: irritability, foggy brain, and fatigue. You might even feel fluish. However, within a week your symptoms will subside. After this, never eat wheat or more than 10 grams of sugar in one serving again, or your addiction will start all over again. (Ugh.)

Day 3

1. Eliminate Processed Foods

Do not eat processed foods from boxes and bags.

2. Implement Healthy Eating Guidelines

Make 50 percent of your food fresh and raw. Follow the Healthy Eating Guidelines provided in appendix 5.

Add digestive enzymes to your meals if you're having trouble digesting food (belching, indigestion). A health-food store attendant can provide advice regarding which digestive enzyme to purchase.

. . .

Days 4 and 5 (Saturday and Sunday)

Continue to implement all the steps listed on day one through three as you proceed.

1. Rest

Focus on you. Rest, read, pray, and ask God to help you to succeed.

2. Use the Sword of the Spirit

Now is the time to fight the thief Jesus spoke of in John 10:10, for Satan wants you to fail: "The thief's purpose is to steal, kill and destroy. My purpose is to give life in all its fullness" (John 10:10 TLB).

Fight the thief with the sword of the Spirit—the Word of God. Write verses on index cards or put them on the notes app on your smartphone. Use verses that will remind you of the help God provides in any struggles you may be facing at this point, such as Philippians 4:13: "For I can do everything through Christ, who gives me strength." Every time you get the urge to go back to your old eating habits, speak the verse out loud to cut the demonic influence out of your life. Our spiritual nature needs to be addressed as well as our physical.

Day 6

1. Start the Anti-Candida Cleanse

Now let's kill the bug in your gut—Candida. Today, start the anti-Candida cleanse you purchased in step 4. If you are not ready to begin this step because you are still experiencing symptoms of withdrawal (headache, exhaustion, irritability, mental fogginess, fluish symptoms), wait a few days until you feel better. Read the instructions on the cleanse package for how to administer it. Initially, I recommend taking the cleanse every other day for the first week to minimize lethargy and headaches. You will feel awful if the dead Candida is not quickly expelled from your colon. To avoid becoming constipated, drink plenty of water. During the second week, begin taking the Candida cleanse every day as recommended.

How long should you stay on the Candida cleanse? The cleanse label provides specific instructions, though it depends on the severity of your Candida overgrowth. Through a colonic irrigation, my therapist found I had a severe Candida infection. I stayed on the cleanse until I finished the bottle—about a month. In fact, I took a second bottle as well. Currently, I go on the cleanse every time I begin having symptoms of a Candida infection (crave carbs and feel fatigued), and I usually stay on the cleanse for one week.

During this cleanse you need frequent bowel movements to eliminate the dead Candida from your colon. If you become constipated, you will get a headache. Prevent a headache by increasing the fiber in your diet through a fiber supplement (which usually comes with your Candida cleanse), water, and raw fruits and vegetables.

The first three days you are on the cleanse, you may not feel well, but after a week you will begin to feel better than you have in a long time. You are just about to get the life back Jesus wants you to experience—one that is abundant and full.

Regarding bowel movements (BM), humans should have at least one a day, if not two, when you are not on a cleanse. When my sister started the cleanse, she had four BMs in one day. She had a lot of fecal matter built up in her colon. Think of a colon like a pipe with sludge built up on the inside. A colon could have a half-inch of fecal matter sticking to it. We use Drano to clean out our drain and pipes. The cleanse is kind of like Drano for the colon. This cleanse is milder than a colonoscopy prep. My sister lost a pound that day!

Day 7
1. Get Up and Exercise

If you are still feeling the symptoms of withdrawal, be gentle with yourself by performing a simple form of exercise such as walking or yoga.

It doesn't matter what type of exercise you do just as long as you do it. Walking, jumping rope, lifting weights, or taking a group fitness class like Pilates or water aerobics are a few examples of exercise. After you begin feeling better, try to exercise for twenty minutes three times a week. I found the book *Eat Right 4 Your Type* by Dr. Peter

D'Adamo informative regarding the type of activity each blood type is most inclined to enjoy. It was right on for me with yoga, swimming, bicycling, and hiking.

Record the exercise you perform in your journal that you set up in step 2. If you haven't been or aren't exercising, determine why you don't do it more. Is it because you don't have the time or you're too tired? Is there any type of exercise you enjoy? Figure out what you like to do and put it on your calendar. Ask a family member, friend, or neighbor to join you on a regular basis, so you encourage each other to keep up this beneficial habit.

If you previously consumed high-sugar products, the fluctuations in your blood sugar may have caused lethargy, especially when blood-sugar levels plummeted. As you remove these products from your diet, at first you will become even more tired, but after a week or two, your energy level will increase. At that time, you can explore additional exercise activities. Is there a type of physical endeavor you enjoyed when you were younger? Maybe it's time to try it again.

Recently, I joined a Facebook group that schedules hikes on Saturday mornings. I enjoy meeting new people and conversing as we walk in a unique setting each week. The time flies while walking with friends. Do you have someone you could walk with? Sharing workouts with another person makes it more enjoyable and adds accountability.

I love to swim because when I am under the water, it feels like a different world. If you find an activity you enjoy, it becomes a pleasure instead of a burden. Figure out what you like to do, carve out the time, and do it!

Irrefutable evidence exists that regular physical activity prevents numerous chronic diseases such as diabetes, cancer, obesity, depression, hypertension, osteoporosis, osteoarthritis, and cardiovascular disease.[1] In fact, the most physically active people are the ones with the lowest risk of contracting these chronic diseases.[2] So get out and do whatever physical activity you appreciate. What matters is that you get moving.

Two months after my sister started this lifestyle change, she joined a gym. The trainer set up her routine for the machines and weights. As she tried different group fitness classes, she found Zumba was too fast for her, but she enjoyed the pace of yoga.

I teach Christian yoga. For years I could've found an excuse to not go to the gym--it's raining, I'm tired--you get the picture. But because I taught the class I had to show up. Join an exercise class where you have accountability (you paid for the class, or you have someone to hold you accountable to attend).

The gentle Christian yoga class I teach is called Scripture Yoga™. I created two DVDs, "God's Mighty Angels" and "What the Bible Says about Prayer," and two books, *Scripture Yoga* and *Yoga for Beginners.* Seniors love my class because it improves their flexibility. I have clients who attend up into their eighties. If you desire gentle exercise, yoga may do the trick. Check out my website at ChristianYoga.com and Facebook page at Facebook.com/ScriptureYoga.

Mindfulness exercises such as yoga and meditation train a person to pay attention to cravings without reacting to them. The idea is to ride out the wave of intense desire. As a person becomes more mindful she notices why she wants to indulge. Meditation quiets the part of the brain that can lead to a loop of obsession.[3]

Day 8 and Beyond

You are well on your way to changing your lifestyle, but more than that you will change your life for the better. Your health, mood, and energy level will improve. Each week you will lose weight, and the body God gave you will heal itself of many ailments.

As your body heals some diseases can be reversed, you will be able to reduce or eliminate medications because you will no longer suffer from the maladies these medications were treating. However, before stopping any prescription medication be sure to consult with your physician.

Improvement in your vitality will allow you to experience activities you were not able to be involved in before. Overall your well-being and emotional countenance will become revitalized. You are in the process of getting your life back, the one that God wants you to enjoy to its fullest.

PLAN FOR PITFALLS

No one is perfect. You will have days when you eat sugar, wheat, or processed foods. That's okay. This happens to everyone; don't let it discourage you. Share your feelings with your accountability/prayer partner. Pray together. Share with your online group if you joined one. Write about your feelings, obstacles, and victories in your journal. Changing the way you eat will be a challenging journey, but one you can conquer.

Every morning spend time with God and plan your day. Determine your menu for the day and what temptations you might encounter. What time of the day would you most likely engage in unhealthy eating? Decide how you will fight food temptation for that specific day. Select a scripture verse and begin the day by reciting it out loud.

When you recognize temptation, remove yourself from the area containing the food, and record the trigger in your journal. Also, write down five reasons why you do not want to eat the food. Put the timer on for ten minutes and spend that time with God. Some strategies for resisting temptation include: pray, go for a walk, recite your Bible verse, call your prayer partner, drink two glasses of water, listen to praise music and start praising God, or utilize other helpful strategies that you develop (see appendix 10 for a list of Food Addiction Battle Strategies). Also, think about how far you have come in overcoming your food addiction and whether you want to experience the withdrawal symptoms again.

If you relapse, get up, brush the dust off yourself, and start again. Realize what triggered your cravings. Was it your emotions? In your journal, keep track of what you ate, why you ate it, what triggered you to eat it, and what you might do the next time you are tempted. *It is vital you record every single time you binge.* Confess your sin to God, and his mercies are new every morning (Lamentations 3:22–23). Ask him to help you do better next time.

Were you tempted by something you saw on TV? If yes, don't watch the commercials. Was it food someone else in your family ate? If yes, ask them not to eat it in front of you. Ask them to store the tempting food products somewhere else in the house. Through journaling, you can identify your triggers and learn how to avoid them.

It is a normal process for people to stay the course and fall off the wagon and binge. This cycle continues to repeat itself, but as you continue to turn to God and rely on his mighty strength, slowly but surely, you will gain control of your body, mind, and spirit.

The changes in your eating habits are a lifelong lifestyle journey so you can live the abundant life Jesus wants you to experience. Not a life filled with disease and unwanted, unhealthy symptoms.

BINDING THE STRONG MAN IN YOUR LIFE

To master addictions, I created the Five-Step Binding the Strong Man Plan. My family had a history of alcoholism, and I did not want to pass this on to my children. I enjoyed consuming alcohol. In fact, I turned to it to relieve my stress instead of God. Alcohol was my spiritual stronghold. A stronghold is something you turn to instead of God. Through using this plan, I tied up the strong man of addiction and kicked him out of my life.

This five-step plan should help a person with any addiction, including food. Before beginning this plan, let's look at God's advice in the Bible in two different translations:

How can anyone enter a strong man's house and carry off his possessions unless he first ties up the strong man? Then he can rob his house.

Matthew 12:29 (NIV)

One cannot rob Satan's kingdom without first binding Satan. Only then can his demons be cast out!

Matthew 12:29 (TLB)

I did not fully understand this verse initially, so I researched its meaning. Adam Clark's commentary states, "Men, through sin, become the very house and dwelling place of Satan (*probably to one of his demons*), having of their own accord surrendered themselves to this unjust possessor; for whoever gives up his soul to sin gives it up to the devil. It is Jesus, and Jesus alone, who can deliver from the power of this bondage. When Satan is cast out, Jesus purifies and dwells in the heart" (emphasis mine).[4] In other words, when a person surrenders to a specific sin over and over again, he or she becomes the dwelling place of an evil spirit. Theological controversy exists about whether Christians can be possessed or only oppressed.

Some examples of spirits of addiction include: alcohol, cigarettes, caffeine, drugs, food, sex, pornography, masturbation, TV, video games, shopping/buying, gambling, etc., but there are also spirits of fear, worry, greed, anxiety, depression, loneliness, unworthiness, unforgiveness, hatred/anger, etc. All of these can be strongholds in one's life.

How can you tell when a particular spirit is a strong man in your life? You can recognize it when these manifestations cause a desire so overpowering you succumb to the temptation over and over again. Even when you don't want to, you can't help it—it's like a battle raging inside you.

Paul struggled with sin as indicated in Romans 7:14-15, "The trouble is with me, for I am all too human, a slave to sin. I don't really understand myself, for I want to do what is right, but I don't do it. Instead, I do what I hate."

What drove you to eat poorly? Is it a food addiction, emotional issue with food, spiritual bondage, Candida infection, or lack of understanding about which foods negatively impact your health? Record the answer to this question in your journal.

When people yield themselves to a vice often enough, the power of the sin becomes attached to them, and they soon become driven by it. They no longer merely think a thought; the thought commands them. That is a strong man—a spirit that attaches itself to your being in a strong way. It has a stronghold in your life, and it won't let go.

Remember, "We are not fighting against people made of flesh and blood, but against persons without bodies—the evil rulers of the unseen world, those mighty satanic beings and great evil princes of darkness who rule this world; and against huge numbers of wicked spirits in the spirit world" (Ephesians 6:12 TLB). Even though the fight gets intense, with God we can overcome any temptation.

Since there is a war going on in the spiritual realm, we may be exposed to an evil spirit at some time in our lives. No one is immune from demonic harassment. If you get to the point where you can identify the strong man for who and what he is, you can do something about it. More specifically, you can bind the strong man who comes against you, as stated in Matthew 12:29.

To be quite frank, what I am addressing is whether you have an evil spirit of addiction oppressing you. Have you taken the food addiction test? Do you think the craving for refined carbohydrates is merely a Candida infection or is there a possibility of a spiritual component?

If you think your food addiction has a spiritual connection, because you feel helpless to control the way you eat, the five-step plan will help you fight domination by an evil spirit. This plan will help you take your life back! See appendix 8 for a summary of this plan.

Five-Step Binding the Strong Man Plan
1. Name what controls you.
Name the thing controlling you—food addiction, anxiety, eating disorder, depression, etc.—whatever it may be, and declare (out loud) Jesus Christ is your Lord in its place![5]

For me, it was the desire to drink alcohol. I liked the way it made me feel. I identified that this desire was a generational curse handed down from my grandfather to my father and from him to me. I wanted it to stop. I did not want to hand this curse down to my children. I recognized alcohol became a stronghold in my life because I turned to a drink to handle my stress rather than turning to God. Turning to alcohol happened over and over again until I used the steps in this plan to tie up the strong man of alcohol addiction in my life.

Stand up to the evil spirit who brought bondage into your life by saying, "Evil spirit, you won't lord over me nor entice me through (insert your addiction) anymore. Jesus is my Lord!" A person obtains spiritual power and authority through Christ. Declare that the spiritual powers of darkness will not have lordship over your life. They will not rule you, govern your behavior, capture your thought life, nor lead you into temptation and sin because "the one who is in you is greater than the one who is in the world" (1 John 4:4 NIV).

"For when Satan, strong and fully armed, guards his palace, it is safe—until someone stronger and better armed attacks and overcomes him and strips him of his weapons and carries off his belongings."

Luke 11:21–22 (TLB)

Get ready, for *you are capable of evicting the addiction strong man in your life*. If you accepted Jesus as your Lord and Savior (see appendix 7 to find out how), the Holy Spirit lives within you and the Spirit is stronger than Satan. Day after day, declare out loud that Jesus reigns as the Lord of your life—not your addiction.

What food problems have been with you since childhood? My sister was hooked on candy and sugary foods since a child. For me, it was the generational bondage of alcoholism. Take some time with

God and record in your journal what instances from your past resulted in the way you eat today.

2. Submit yourself completely to God.

"Submit yourself to God, resist the devil and he will flee from you." James 4:7 (NIV)

There is a secret to resisting the devil—you must first submit yourself to God. How in the world do you do that? In my experience, you no longer do your will but God's will by submitting your life to him. For me, it was not without a fight.

I finally recognized the Holy Spirit's desires within me after I read *The Purpose Driven Life*. The Spirit's wishes felt like my conscience. After this recognition, God began nudging me to grow with simple requests like spending more time with him.

At first after I struggled with wanting my way, not Gods, but I recognized what was going on, and repented. Now when I recognize the Holy Spirit's leading in my life, I try to obey. I am not perfect, therefore, I repent when I realize I did not submit my will to God, and I ask him to help me do better the next time.

If you are a food addict, after binging, ask God to forgive you and help you not to binge the next time. Record your experience in your journal. Once you ask for forgiveness, God chooses not to remember your sins, as indicated in Hebrews 8:12: "And I will be merciful to them in their wrongdoings, and I will remember their sins no more" (TLB). Don't fret over a stumble. Get up and try again using this Five-Step Binding the Strong Man Plan.

3. Use the name of Jesus.

Jesus told his disciples, "Look, I have given you authority over all the power of the enemy" (Luke 10:19). If you are a disciple of Jesus (see appendix 7 to find out how) you can accept the authority he gave you.

In the book of Acts, the apostles healed and worked miracles in the name of Jesus. Use Jesus's name as Peter did in Acts 3:6: "in the name of Jesus Christ of Nazareth, walk" (TLB). Using the name of Jesus is key to binding the strong man because then you operate under Jesus's authority.

Picture a person tied in ropes. That's the way a spiritual strong man afflicts his victim. However, if you declare Jesus is Lord over your life, not the strong man (addiction), and use Jesus's name, you are under his authority. Then the ropes, tied around you by the evil spirit, break. Eventually, the spiritual ropes loosen and fall off. Next, comes the moment to take action by tying the strong man through binding him with the Word of God.

4. Use the Word of God.

"For when Satan, strong and fully armed, guards his palace, it is safe—until someone stronger and better armed attacks and overcomes him and strips him of his weapons and carries off his belongings."

Luke 11:21–22 TLB

The Holy Spirit inside of you is stronger than Satan and his demons. By using the name of Jesus, you are not only under his authority but you can speak with his authority. You are much better armed than Satan. Now is the time to stand up to him, strip him of his weapons, and kick him out of your life through the Word of God!

Say to the strong man, "In the name of Jesus, you won't oppress me anymore. I bind your power in the name of Jesus and by the Word of God."

Search the Bible for a verse that is the opposite of your addiction. A list of verses is provided in appendix 1. Here are two examples:

No discipline is enjoyable while it is happening—it's painful! But afterward there will be a peaceful harvest of right living for those who are trained in this way.

Hebrews 12:11

Dear friends, I warn you as "temporary residents and foreigners" to keep away from worldly desires that wage war against your very souls.

1 Peter 2:11

I used Ephesians 5:18: "Don't drink too much wine, for many evils lie along that path be filled instead with the Holy Spirit and controlled by him." Use the specific scripture you chose to bind the strong man every time he tempts you. Write this verse on an index card and memorize it.

While at a party, I implemented this plan to fight Satan and I won. There was a band, catered food, and an open bar. Oh my! How I wanted a drink, but didn't want one at the same time. The spiritual battle was on. Who would win? I had three fundamental factors on my side:

1. I had sworn God was the Lord of my life—I was not going to turn to alcohol but to God.

2. I submitted my will to God.

3. I memorized the verse about not drinking too much wine.

The desire to consume an alcoholic beverage at the open bar came upon me again and again that evening. At that time, I had no idea an evil spirit bound me in spiritual chains that went as far back as my childhood. To fight my addiction, I recited Ephesians 5:18 to bombard the strong man over and over again.

Praise God, I did not succumb to the temptation to drink. When I left the party, I felt like I fought the devil and won! Through the power of the Holy Spirit, Jesus's authority, and the Word of God, I bound that evil spirit—the strong man.

Luke 11:22 states the strong man was stripped of his weapons and his belongings were carried off. Matthew 12:29 asserts when Satan was bound his demons could be cast out. Well, the evil spirit that gave me the desire to drink was cast out of my life. Now the urge to drink alcohol is no longer an uncontrollable temptation since the evil spirit was stripped of his weapons.

After you tie up the strong man with the Word of God—ignore him. He will try to hobble after you because he doesn't give up easily. If he did, he wouldn't be a strong man. Remember, the next time you are tempted, you're facing a critical moment. When you give him (the spirit of addiction) your attention by drinking, eating sugary foods, worrying—whatever addiction it was—you are, in effect, untying the strong man.

To help you continue ignoring the strong man, recite your opposing Bible verse and ask God for help.

5. Praise God and practice gratitude.

When you praise God and thank him for his blessings, the strong man won't hang around. Don't be satisfied with binding the strong man and walking away—punish him.

Fill your mind, heart, and body with the Spirit of God by putting the right things in your spirit. Listen to praise music; read the Bible and pray; memorize scripture; attend church, Sunday school, or a Bible study. Also, start doing more to help others. Performing acts of service and helping others fills your heart with honorable feelings and humility. Every day, write in your journal about all you can praise God for and thank him.

When you embrace a mind-set of gratitude, dopamine releases in your brain. Remember that dopamine, the feel-good neurohormone, releases when you eat sugar and wheat. Instead of getting the positive feeling from a bad habit, get it from a good one—by journaling gratefulness. If you would like to become more grateful, check out my friend's book The Gratitude Journal: A 21 Day Challenge to More Gratitude, Deeper Relationships, and Greater Joy. Next time you want to eat something unhealthy, grab your journal instead.

Beat the strong man by declaring Bible verses out loud. Stomp him into the ground by singing praises to God. I created a worship playlist on my phone, and I listen to it every morning as I get ready for work. Before long, I lift my arms in praise and worship to our almighty God. The devil can't stand to be around someone who worships the Lord.

Become God's warrior by using his mighty unseen weapons. Paul advises, "It is true that I am an ordinary, weak human being, but I don't use human plans and methods to win my battles. I use God's mighty weapons, not those made by men, to knock down the devil's strongholds" (2 Corinthians 10:3–4 TLB). Get ready to knock out and tie up the strong man of addiction in your life. (A simplified version of the Five-Step Binding the Strong Man Plan is included in appendix 8.) You are God's mighty conqueror!

To assist you with the spiritual implications regarding dysfunctional food habits I created Christain Study Guide for 7 Steps to Get Off Sugar and Carbohydrates. This in-depth study goes into more detail regarding accessing God's power, changing your mind-set, and using the armor of God.

TAKING STEP 5: IMPLEMENT THE PHYSICAL AND SPIRITUAL PLANS

Planning is crucial for maintaining this new way of eating you committed to. Take these action steps below as you plan:

1. Implement the Seven-Day Eating Plan listed in appendix 6. Go to SusanUNeal.com/appendix for a printable version of the appendices. Date you will start this plan: _____.

2. Plan for the pitfalls. Print the list of Food Addiction Battle Strategies from appendix 10, and use these strategies as you stumble.

3. Implement the Five-Step Binding the Strong Man Plan and print a copy of the plan.

4. Choose a specific verse to use when the strong man of addiction tempts you. Write the verse on an index card and memorize it.

5. Continue to record pertinent information in your journal such as: what food problems have been with your since childhood, and write about all you can praise God for and thank him.

7 Steps to Get Off Sugar and Carbohydrates:

Step 1. Decide to improve your health through proper nutrition.

Step 2. Acquire a support system and knowledge to help make a lifestyle change.

Step 3. Clean out your pantry and refrigerator by removing unhealthy foods and clean out your emotions.

Step 4. Purchase healthy foods and an anti-Candida cleanse.

Step 5. Plan for the start date to begin changing your eating habits.

Day 1: Drink eight glasses of water per day. Stop eating sugar. Take a probiotic.

Day 2: Stop eating wheat.

Day 3: Do not eat processed foods out of boxes and bags. Make 50 percent of your food be fresh and raw. Follow the Healthy Eating Guidelines provided in appendix 5.

Day 4 and 5: Focus on you. Rest, read, pray, and ask God to give you the willpower to succeed.

Day 6: Begin the anti-Candida cleanse.

Day 7: Get up and exercise.

. . .

Five-Step Plan for Binding the Strong Man of addiction in your life.

1. Name your addiction and declare (out loud) that Jesus Christ is your Lord in its place!

2. Submit yourself completely to God.

3. Bind the strong man with the name of Jesus.

4. Use the Word of God to bind the strong man (evil spirit of addiction).

5. Punish the strong man by praising God and being grateful.

6

STEP 6: PREPARE AND EAT FOODS DIFFERENTLY

Decide—>Acquire—>Clean Out—>Purchase—>Plan—>**Prepare—**>Improve

You have decided to change your eating habits, acquired knowledge, cleaned out the pantry, purchased healthy food, and planned the physical and spiritual steps; now it's time to get to work in the kitchen. In step 6, we will *prepare* for eating in a healthier way, with a suggested weekly menu. Post your menu on the refrigerator, so you know what you planned to cook for each meal during the week. Appendix 4 is full of recipes.

Cooking from scratch is important. For example, do not buy garlic already minced in a jar. You have no idea how old it is. The nutrients from fruits and vegetables begin to break down as soon as you cut them. Instead, mince a fresh clove of garlic.

It might take longer to cook from scratch, but the food will be more nutritious and low in sugar. Also, you will save time and money with less trips to the doctor. Your health is worth it. Your family will appreciate the time you invest into preparing healthy, delicious meals.

Make the transition from eating convenience foods, such as processed foods or eating out, to cooking at home. It doesn't have to be difficult. When Adam and Eve were in the garden of Eden, they picked a fruit or vegetable and ate it. Pretend you are in God's garden that he created for you and dream up what you could prepare. Create a salad with an avocado or nuts (protein). Load a sliced green apple with almond butter. Dip fresh vegetables into a healthy dip like guacamole or hummus. Blend a fruit smoothie with kale or spinach. Bake a large sweet potato—it is very filling. Simple meals work just as well as complicated, complex dishes.

God made you in his image, and he prizes and loves you. You are worthy of the time and effort it takes to invest in yourself. Choose to put yourself higher on your list of priorities. If you do, you will do a better job of living out the life God created for you.

TIPS FOR A HEALTHIER LIFESTYLE

The following tips should assist you to successfully make healthy lifestyle changes. Simple hints like drinking plenty of water or eating only until you are full will help you be more prepared, especially when it comes to choosing healthy foods when eating out.

Only Eat Until You're Full

As you prepare to eat healthier, one positive change you can make is to notice the sensation of fullness as you eat. Some individuals may not be in touch with that feeling anymore. Focus on recognizing when you are full so you do not overeat. You may have to change some of your mealtime habits as well. Eat slowly, chew your food thoroughly, and pay attention to how the food tastes. As you learn to enjoy the taste of foods in their purest form, you'll begin to look for more ways to prepare meals with the variety of amazing foods God created for our health.

When you eat processed foods, versus meals you prepare from scratch, it takes a larger quantity of the refined product to fill your stomach because these foods do not contain the original food's fiber. Think of crushing a bag of chips versus shredding carrots and celery. The fresh vegetables will satiate your hunger with a smaller volume.

When you eat foods closer to their form at harvest, you will become full with smaller portions. The feeling of fullness stays with you for a longer period too, so you don't need to snack as much. By following this simple lifestyle change, you will eat a smaller quantity of food loaded with vitamins, minerals, fiber, and all the nutrients the human body needs—the way God intended for you to eat.

Pay attention to portion size. Think of your stomach as the size of your fist—before it is stretched out by food. Put less food on your plate than you think you will eat. Use a smaller plate. As soon as you feel full, stop eating and put the timer on for five minutes. When the timer rings, you shouldn't feel hungry anymore since it takes a little while for your brain to recognize your stomach reached its capacity. If you stop eating at the first sign you feel the sensation of fullness, in five minutes your brain receptors catch up with the feeling in your stomach.

Eating Out

Realistically, you won't be able to prepare meals at home all the time. Our lives are busy and many days we are unable to eat at home, so on occasion we will eat out. Let's first address fast food. We need to use drive-throughs when traveling or in a hurry. Most fast-food restaurants provide a selection of healthy options to choose from, such as a fresh salad with raw ingredients. However, be sure to use either no dressing or as small a portion as you can. If you use more than one fast-food package of salad dressing, you just made your positive eating choice into a negative one.

Healthy eating choices at a dine-in restaurant are a vegetable plate, fish, or chicken. First, check the menu for the ingredients in your meal choice, and make sure you ask for your food to be served in the healthiest way: no sauces and baked or gilled instead of fried. When your food arrives, the serving size may be substantial. Therefore, when served a large plate of food, before you begin eating, determine how much you will eat to prevent overeating. You might even ask for a to-go container at the beginning of your meal to store what you will not eat at this meal. It is difficult to stop unless you establish boundaries before you begin eating delicious foods.

Drink Your Daily Water Intake

If you get hungry in between meals, drink two glasses of water. Water usually curbs your appetite. Most people mistake the feeling of thirst for hunger. Our bodies desperately need water to flush out the toxins and prevent dehydration. You also will have more energy when you drink an adequate amount of water.

My sister found it challenging to incorporate drinking eight glasses of water into her daily routine, especially on an empty stomach. It is best not to drink during meals because the fluid dilutes gastric juices that break down food. She previously drank sweet tea and sodas instead of water and this increased her sugar consumption. I suggested she drink two glasses of water before breakfast, two before lunch, two midafternoon, and two before dinner (my recommendation in steps 4 and 5).

I stop drinking fluids at 6 pm, so I don't have to get up to go to the bathroom as much at night. Try not to forget about drinking all day long and then consume a lot of water after dinner. Getting up in the middle of the night to go to the bathroom disrupts sleep. Plan when you will consume your eight glasses of water during the day.

Follow the Healthy Eating Guidelines

As you prepare your weekly menu, keep in mind these Healthy Eating Guidelines from step 4 (purchase) listed below and also in appendix 5:

- Buy organic fruits, vegetables, and meats.

- About 50 percent of your food should be fresh, organic vegetables.
- Eat one fresh, raw serving of a low-glycemic fruit per day. Low-glycemic fruits include green apples, berries, cherries, pears, plums, and grapefruit.
- Do not always eat cooked foods. Eat a couple of servings of raw vegetables every day. Eat a salad for lunch with nuts, meat, or an avocado. When eating out, order a salad or coleslaw as sides since both are raw.
- Plan for 25 percent of your food to be an animal or vegetable protein such as beans, nuts, and lean meats. Fish is especially nutritious.
- A variety of different nuts and seeds are excellent sources of protein, minerals, and essential fatty acids.
- Eat nontraditional grains such as quinoa, amaranth, pearled barley, and oats.

MEAL PLANNING

To help my sister on this journey to change her eating habits I provided her with examples of healthy meals. The following daily meal categories include a list of appropriate healthy food options for your menu planning and shopping lists.

Breakfast

- oatmeal with pecans and cinnamon
- pancakes made with almond flour (A link for this recipe: Pinterest.com/SusanUNeal/breakfast/)
- quinoa with a smashed banana, almond milk, and walnuts
- scrambled eggs with hash browns
- omelet with green onions, red peppers, and mushrooms
- berries with plain Greek yogurt
- chia parfait with fruit

- homemade granola with berries and/or Greek yogurt
- hash browns with onions, peppers, and a sliced avocado on top
- mashed avocado with two fried eggs on top
- pancakes made with two eggs and one smashed banana

Lunch

- a salad or vegetable plate, if eating out
- romaine lettuce wrap sandwich with any meat or vegetable
- cucumber sandwich—cut a cucumber in half and load it with meat (not lunch meat) and veggies
- salad with fish, chicken, nuts, or avocado
- baked potato bar with olive oil, broccoli, scallions, sunflower seeds
- guacamole or hummus with sliced vegetables
- whole avocado and an heirloom tomato
- baked sweet potato with butter, cinnamon, and honey

Snack

- sliced green apple with almond or cashew butter
- berries with whipped cream made with coconut milk
- raw vegetables with hummus or guacamole
- boiled egg or deviled eggs (made with organic mayonnaise)
- carrots and celery sticks
- berries with slivered almonds
- nuts—raw almonds, pecans, pistachios, macadamia nuts, or cashews
- organic popcorn popped on the stove (not microwave popcorn)

Dinner

- chicken fajitas with guacamole, lettuce, tomato, and avocado on a coconut tortilla wrap (available at health food stores)
- spaghetti with a baked spaghetti squash for the noodles
- steak, mushrooms, green beans with slivered almonds, and a salad
- salmon, sautéed red cabbage, and wild rice
- baked or grilled chicken, quinoa, and sautéed or grilled zucchini and yellow squash
- chili made with lean meat
- fish, salad, and asparagus
- beef stew with potato, carrots, celery, bok choy, and onions
- black bean soup
- fresh field peas with sliced tomatoes, fried okra, and corn pone bread (recipe in appendix 4)
- shrimp fettuccine alfredo with shirataki noodles, and a salad
- roasted whole chicken with onions, potatoes, carrots, and bok choy
- salad with berries, nuts, and seeds

Dessert

- dark chocolate (at least 70 percent chocolate)
- dark chocolate almond cookies (recipe in appendix 4)
- chocolate nut clusters (see directions in the section Curb the Sweettooth)
- dark chocolate–covered strawberries

- one dried date to seven pecan halves (be careful, as dates are high in sugar)

MENU PLANNING

If you haven't planned your menu already, choose a pleasant spot (outside, by a fire, coffee shop), to plan your menu and corresponding grocery list. This may take up to an hour, but is well worth your time and effort. Use this book, another healthy cookbook, or an app on your phone to find recipes. I have a provided a list of recipe resources in step 2.

I list what I plan to cook for breakfast, lunch, dinner, and snack for every day of the week. As I choose a recipe, I put the corresponding ingredients that I need on my grocery list. For years, as my children were growing up, I posted on their chalkboard what the menu was for every day of the week. Everyone in the family knew what I would be serving.

I cooked on Sunday and Monday and listed leftovers (from Sunday) to be served on Tuesday. Wednesday we all ate at church, and Thursday I served leftovers from Monday. Two nights of cooking took care of four meals. To liven up a leftover, I would cook one new item (such as a vegetable) to be served with the previous meal, and this new item gave the meal new interest.

I created a standard grocery list for the store I used. For me, it was Walmart. To create this list, initially I walked through the store and either wrote or dictated into my smartphone notes app the items I normally purchased on those aisles. For example, I would start in the refrigerated section and would include eggs, butter, coconut milk, and non-dairy yogurt on the list for that aisle. Then I proceeded to the next aisle, cleaning supplies and paper products. I listed Clorox wipes, toilet paper, napkins, paper towels, paper plates, etc. At home, I typed out this list based on each grocery store aisle and the products I normally purchased. It took work to create this list, but it has stream-lined my grocery store planning for years.

Each week I printed a fresh new list and my family knew that if we ran out of an item, they circled it on the list or wrote it out. I made a rule to guide us—if it wasn't on the list it didn't get purchased. I put the responsibility on them, not all on me.

Every week I made some sort of fresh, raw salad (broccoli salad, beet salad, coleslaw, salad with lettuce) and I ate that for my lunch. For my children's lunch boxes, I tried to include one fresh fruit and vegetable. When they wanted a fruit roll-up, I explained that I was giving them something better by giving them a real piece of fruit (their choice) because it was loaded with the natural vitamins and minerals that God put into the fruit to nourish our bodies. My children learned the importance of whole God-given foods.

After you plan your menu and purchase all those groceries, it is time to start cooking healthy homemade meals. If you need help with planning your menu, join my blog at HealthLivingSeriesBlog.com where I post menus and corresponding grocery lists.

PREPARE TO COOK

As I planned my menu I also designated who would be cooking the meal. I assigned each of my children a night to assist me in the kitchen at least one time per week. Mealtime preparation can be a great opportunity for bonding.

Each morning I checked my menu posted on the refrigerator to determine if I needed to defrost any frozen items. I determined the time to serve our meal and began cooking one hour prior to that time. Most meals required some sort of chopping of vegetables, so if another family member assisted me, I had them do this job. When cooking alone, I turned on my praise music and enjoyed creating a colorful, delicious meal. I felt I was providing my family with a beautiful love offering.

I always cooked more than was needed so I would have enough food left over for future meals. If I was taking the time to prepare a healthy meal from scratch, I wanted to make sure that my efforts were fully utilized. I had everyone serve themselves, and whoever did not assist me in cooking had kitchen clean-up duty.

CURB YOUR SWEET TOOTH

Surprisingly, taste buds change when you eat natural foods. As you eliminate sugar from your diet, your pallet changes, and the healthy snacks listed below will seem sweet to you. When the craving for sugar arises, I eat one of these nutritious snacks (this list is also provided in appendix 9):

- Slice a green apple, which is low in sugar, and add almond or cashew butter to each slice. It tastes sweet; conversely, the almond butter is high in protein. Both the apple and nut butter provide fiber and fill me up.
- Melt 70-percent dark chocolate in a pan on the stove and add different types of nuts until well coated with the chocolate. Place mounds of nut clusters on wax paper. After an hour they harden. Keep in an airtight container on the counter or refrigerator for a week. Nuts contain fiber and are filling.
- Sparingly eat one date along with seven pecan halves. Dates are high in natural sugar, so you only need a smidgen to attain the sweetness. Don't eat too many dates, but instead fill up on the pecans, which are high in protein.
- I grow fruit trees in my yard, so from June through December I pick fresh blueberries, apples, grapes, pears, and oriental persimmons. I eat one serving of fruit each day either for breakfast or as an afternoon snack.
- Curb sweet cravings by adding a teaspoon of raw, unfiltered, unpasteurized apple cider vinegar in a cup of water with a couple of drops of stevia.

Learning a new skill is difficult at the beginning, but with time, your new eating habits will become routine. Recognize you can say no to the voice in your head that demands unhealthy food. Instead of giving in to this voice, put the timer on for fifteen minutes to delay food gratification. Training yourself to wait before you eat will help you gain better self-control. During that time preoccupy yourself by writing in your journal.

JOURNAL

In step 2 and appendix 3, I recommended that you purchase the *Healthy Living Journal* or write the following items in your journal any time you eat:

1. The time you eat.
2. Why you are about to eat. Are you hungry, bored, angry? Is it just "time to eat" or are you with others who are having a meal?
3. If you feel a strong emotion related to this consumption of food, record the emotion.
4. What you ate and drank, including quantity.
5. How you feel after you ate? Satisfied or stuffed?
6. After you eat, record how the food makes you feel regarding your energy level and clarity of mind.
7. When waking up in the morning, how do you feel? See if there is a pattern of eating high-sugar-content foods and feeling sluggish the next morning.
8. What are you grateful for today?
9. Prayer requests to God.
10. Exercise—type and length of time.
11. Number of glasses of water you drink and when. Did you drink on an empty stomach?
12. Every time you binge, record: what you ate, why you ate it, what triggered you to eat it, and what you might do the next time you are tempted.

As you write this information, determine if there is a pattern to your behavior as it relates to eating. Do you eat because you are hungry? If not, why do you want to eat? Do you have at least three hours in between meals? It takes three to four hours for your previous meal to digest, and your stomach to empty. Change your mind-set from immediate gratification to thinking about how this food will make you feel and whether it will nourish the temple of the Holy Spirit.

Continue to journal for the first three months as you make this lifestyle change. You may continue journaling longer if you feel it is helping you achieve your goals. However, as you improve your eating habits, you may only need to journal if and when you binge (see #12 above).

SPIRITUAL PREPARATION

You prepared the kitchen by cleaning out the pantry and refrigerator, planned the menu, purchased food, and prepared meals. However, you also need to prepare spiritually because the enemy will attack. Post the Five-Step Binding the Strong Man Plan from appendix 8 on your refrigerator or bathroom mirror and use it when tempted to overeat unhealthy foods.

To overcome a spiritual battle with food, I recommend the study *Christian Study Guide for 7 Steps to Get Off Sugar and Carbohydrates*. It goes into renewing the mind by bringing every thought captive to Jesus Christ. Whether you do this study by yourself or with a group, it will help you go more in-depth to resolve the spiritual component of a food addiction.

You are in a battle, so you need to develop a strategy. From journaling, have you identified your food triggers? Do you have a plan for how to reduce those triggers? Have you told yourself lies that justify inappropriate eating? Journal those lies. Replace those lies with the Word of God.

I challenge you to learn one new scripture verse per week. Choose the verse, write it on an index card, and memorize it. Step 2 includes tactics to help you memorize Bible verses. When you choose to learn God's Word it will affect you in positive ways you can't begin to imagine. We are supposed to store his word in our hearts so we can draw upon it when the enemy tells us lies. Store the sword of the Spirit in your mind and you can defeat Satan, and successfully achieve the goals in the contract you wrote to God in step 1.

Develop and document your battle strategies in your *Healthy Living Journal*. Some of your Food Addiction Battle Strategies (listed in appendix 10) should include:

1. Record pertinent information in your journal.
2. Find a specific Bible verse to oppose your food issue and write it on an index card. Keep it with you until you memorize it. Speak the verse out loud every time you feel the urge to eat unhealthy foods.
3. Ask a friend to be your accountability and prayer partner.
4. Join a Christian weight loss program or an online food addiction program.
5. Determine food triggers and eliminate them.
6. Implement the Five Steps to Binding the Strong Man Plan:
7. Name the thing controlling you—your food addiction, anxiety, eating disorder, depression, etc.—whatever it may be, and declare (out loud) Jesus Christ is your Lord in its place!
8. Submit yourself completely to God.
9. Bind the strong man (evil spirit of addiction) with the name of Jesus.
10. Use the Word of God to bind the strong man.
11. Punish the strong man by praising God.

Do you have an accountability/prayer partner, yet? Acquiring a support system is integral to successfully make this lifestyle change. Have you joined a Christian weight loss program or one of the online food addiction programs? A list of these programs is provided in appendix 2. If you need to, reread step 2 about how to create your support system.

When you binge, be sure to journal afterward—every single time. There is a Binge Eating Tracker chart in the *Healthy Living Journal*. Figure out what you told yourself that validated why it was okay to eat the item. Then go through the Five Steps to Binding the Strong Man Plan (appendix 8). If you journal and implement this five-step plan every time you binge, you will experience success. Retraining your mind is like disciplining a child; consistency is vital to conformity.

Don't tell yourself lies such as "a little bit of food with sugar will curb my appetite." Instead, sugar will open up the floodgate for you to binge on that sweet food item. My hairdresser asked me how I was able to not eat sugary foods or refined carbohydrates. She said she eliminates these foods for a while, but as soon as she eats one item with sugar, she starts craving it all over again. She is completely right. Therefore, do not eat anything with more than 10 grams of sugar in one serving, or 24 grams for a woman or 36 grams for a man per day. (Check out the list of natural sweet snacks to Curb the Sweet Tooth in appendix 9.)

If you tell yourself lies to break your eating rules and eat what you regret, I recommend you get the app "I Deserve a Donut and Other Lies That Make You Eat" by Barb Raveling. Some of the lies this app evaluates include:

"I'll never be skinny so I might as well eat."

"I deserve this."

"I need this."

You can't serve God to your fullest if your body doesn't function well. The Holy Spirit inside of you is holy, so you should honor the body that carries the Spirit. First Corinthians 6:19–20 states, "Don't you realize that your body is the temple of the Holy Spirit, who lives in you and was given to you by God? You do not belong to yourself, for God bought you with a high price. So you must honor God with your body." *You honor God with your body through making this lifestyle change to improve your health.*

Scripture indicates you are a priest to serve God: "To him who loves us and has freed us from our sins by his blood, and has made us to be a kingdom and priests to serve his God and Father" (Revelation 1:6 NIV). If you are overweight or develop a chronic disease, it will be hard to fulfill your privilege and responsibility to the Lord. Of course, not all diseases can be cured by proper nutrition. However, diabetes, obesity, high blood pressure, cardiovascular disease, and cancer can be affected, positively or negatively, by your diet.

Changing your eating habits for the better reminds me of accepting Christ as your Lord and Savior. Many people choose not to accept Jesus's precious gift. Will you choose to accept this lifestyle change to improve your health? The decision is yours.

You should feel great about the steps you have taken to improve your health and well-being. I am proud of you and so is God. You are well on your way to achieving your goals.

TAKING STEP 6: PREPARE

This step helps you prepare for a new way of eating not only in your menu and meal plans but in spiritual preparation for the changes you are making. Take the action steps listed below:

1. Plan your menu for the week and post it on the refrigerator.
2. Create a standardized grocery list that you can print out every week when planning your menu.
3. Go grocery shopping.
4. Prepare healthy meals from scratch using the Healthy Eating Guidelines in appendix 5. For a a a printable version of the appendix go to SusanUNeal.com/appendix.
5. Pay attention to:
6. Portion control
7. Water intake
8. Eat fresh and raw items at fast-food restaurants.
9. Use techniques to curb your sweet tooth (see appendix 9).
10. Continue to record pertinent information in your journal.

Have you identified your food triggers? Do you have a plan for how to reduce those triggers? Have you told yourself lies that justify inappropriate eating? Journal those lies. Replace those lies with the Word of God.

11. Memorize one scripture verse per week. Choose the verse, write it on an index card, and memorize it.

12. Download the app "I Deserve a Donut and Other Lies That Make You Eat" by Barb Raveling.

7 Steps to Get Off Sugar and Carbohydrates:

Step 1. Decide to improve your health through proper nutrition.

Step 2. Acquire a support system and knowledge to help make a lifestyle change.

Step 3. Clean out your pantry and refrigerator by removing unhealthy foods and clean out your emotions.

Step 4. Purchase healthy foods and an anti-Candida cleanse.

Step 5. Plan for the start date to begin changing your eating habits.

Step 6. Prepare and eat foods differently than you did before.

7

STEP 7: IMPROVE YOUR HEALTH

Decide—>Acquire—>Clean   out—>Purchase—>Plan—>Prepare—
>**Improve**

When you take the steps outlined in this book, your health, and energy levels *improve* because you eat healthy foods that nourish your body. After a week of being off sugar, cravings for it and for carbohydrates cease. Understanding your food triggers helps you stay away from unhealthy foods. Now you need to continue this lifestyle change for the rest of your life, never turning back to your old eating habits.

Don't make your expectations too high. Remember the 80/20 rule: if you improve your eating 80 percent of the time, you will improve your diet. This lifestyle change is not an all-or-nothing situation. If you don't follow the dietary guidelines provided in this book 100 percent of the time, don't have the mind-set that you failed. Instead, give yourself grace as God does. Try to do well, but if you don't eat correctly 20 percent of the time, that's okay. It's probably better than the way you ate before.

Expect to stumble. You will not change your eating habits entirely. Don't get discouraged when you do not meet your expectations.

Making this lifestyle change is difficult, but with the help of Christ, you can succeed.

GIVE YOURSELF GRACE

Many people get into a cycle of diets. They do well for a while, but when they make a mistake, they feel terrible about themselves, as if they failed. So they return to unhealthy eating habits.

An all-or-nothing attitude is perilous. If you blow your eating guidelines, stop overeating as soon as possible and continue to follow the healthy eating standards for the rest of the day. Just because you slipped doesn't mean you should binge. As with any attempt to improve your life, when you stumble, get up and try again.

Our thought life can sabotage our success. We must change our thought process from negativity and despair to positivity and hope if we are to make the lifestyle changes necessary for a healthy future. We are far from perfect, so don't create expectations of perfection for yourself on this journey. Improvement is the correct mind-set to succeed. Replace any negativity about yourself with God's grace.

Another way to think of grace is to consider how you would advise your best friend who calls you after she binges on food. You would show her grace and help her start again. When you mess up, think about what you would tell her. Don't be so hard on yourself. Understand that at some point you will eat unhealthy foods, and you will overeat. Expect it and move on.

James Allen, a nineteenth-century self-help-movement pioneer, stated, "The greatest discovery of our generation is that human beings can alter their lives by altering their attitudes of mind. As you think, so shall you be."[1] This quote is similar to Proverbs 23:7: "For as he thinks in his heart, so *is* he" (NKJV). What do you think of yourself? Record the answer to this question in your journal. Open up your heart to God and ask him to give you an optimistic mind-set as you give yourself grace.

LET YOUR MISTAKES MOTIVATE YOU

As your diet improves, when you eat foods high in sugar or refined carbohydrates you will feel sluggish. You may not even feel like getting out of bed the next day, and you will be foggy brained. Whereas, if you eat clean, raw foods, your clarity of thought and energy improves.

Every time I slip, I pay for it the next day and that motivates me to eat healthier. I like waking up feeling energized and ready to start my day, rather than feeling groggy. That way, I can serve God to the best of my ability.

Unfortunately, as I write this chapter, I have just overindulged in ice cream (made with coconut milk), and I feel terrible. My blood sugar spiked and then plummeted. I feel drained, and I have a slight headache. I can't concentrate, and I don't feel like working on anything. Do you understand this feeling? I recognize what I did. I will eat better for the rest of today. Tomorrow is a new day, and I will feel better then.

FOOD ADDICTION REVISITED

If you did not previously take the test to determine if you are a food addict, I suggest that you do so. The first step in dealing with any addiction is to acknowledge it. Even if you don't see yourself this way, understanding your body's reaction to foods is crucial for making improvement in your eating and feeling the benefits of a healthier approach to food. Use these links to online quizzes to determine if you are addicted to food: FoodAddicts.org/am-i-a-food-addict and OA.org/newcomers/how-do-i-start/are-you-a-compulsive-overeater/. If you do discover you are a food addict, take the steps necessary to begin to overcome this (see step 1) to improve your lifestyle and food habits.

Addiction rewires the neural circuits in a person's brain. Therefore, the brain assigns a higher value to sugar and wheat than other foods. Subliminal food cues excite the brain's reward system and contribute to a relapse. People fall prey to these unseen triggers. That is why it is imperative to identify what sets off your desire and eliminate the trigger. Similarly, an alcoholic should not go into a bar. As your health improves from eating well, you cannot let down your guard. Recognizing you have a food addiction and avoiding the triggers will keep you in recovery mode and allow you to maintain this healthier lifestyle.

If you are a food addict and are not able to stop the cycle of addiction with the suggestions in this book, I strongly recommend you use the *Christian Study Guide for 7 Steps to Get Off Sugar and Carbohydrates* or join a twelve-step program along with a corresponding support group. You could also join my closed Facebook group: 7 Steps to Get Off Sugar and Carbohydrates. Appendix 2 includes a list of Christian Weight Loss and Food Addiction Programs.

BENEFITS OF HEALTHY EATING

Whether you are dealing with addiction or not, as you nourish your body with the proper nutrients God intended for you to ingest, your body will begin to heal itself of diabetes, hypertension, headaches, allergies, skin problems, joint pain—the list goes on. Complete healing will take some time, yet some unhealthy symptoms may disappear right away. Also, you will lose weight naturally without starving yourself. Your mental clarity will improve, as will the speed of your thought processes. You will love the new you!

How long will it take to stop struggling with food? To answer that question, you need to determine how long you have had a problem with food. If it is more than a decade, it may take over a year to rewire the pathways of your brain and spiritually tie up the strong man of addiction and kick him out of your life. Don't think of this as an overnight fix. It took a while to get into this condition, and it will take a while to get the healthy you back, so be patient. It took me eight months on the anti-Candida diet to kill the yeast in my colon.

THE PATH TO RECOVERY AND HEALTH

If you have a food addiction, your recovery will not be short or easy, but you can do it. "Because the one who is in you is greater than the one who is in the world" (1 John 4:4 NIV). Through the Holy Spirit inside of you, you are powerful. *God is on your side.* Use his powerful words to fight the enemy.

How do you look at food? Are you using food to comfort and meet an emotional need, or do you think of food as a necessity to keep your body functioning? Have you journaled about this? Do you turn to food to help you deal with the challenges of life? If so, food is your stronghold. A stronghold is something you put before God.

Pray and ask the Lord to help you turn to him instead of food. You need to get to the root cause of your dysfunctional food eating issue so you can heal. Turn to God first to meet your needs, not food. You will need to continue to turn to God over and over again asking for his help to free you from food addiction. Getting off sugar and carbohydrates reminds me of training a child. It takes years and a lot of repetition. But at some point, the child gets it and becomes well behaved, most of the time.

During this journey of change, learn from your mistakes. Have you ever thought, *I'll take one bite and that will satisfy my sugar craving?* If so, you understand that logic never works. You can't take only one bite, because dopamine releases in the brain and causes a physiological response that your self-control cannot manage.[2]

Even before you take the first bite, if you desire the food item, dopamine secretes in the brain. Scientists proved this through MRI imaging of the brains of addicts. Therefore, when you feel the temptation to eat refined carbohydrates, recognize it and use one of your strategies we developed in this book (see Food Addiction Battle Strategies in appendix 10). If you understand what is going on in your brain, you can more effectively fight the temptation.

If you need more guidance, I created the course, 7 Steps to Reclaim Your Health and Optimal Weight (SusanUNeal.com/courses/7-steps-to-get-off-sugar-and-carbs-course). This course will help you figure out and resolve the root cause of your inappropriate eating habits. One solved, taming your appetite is much easier. I show you how you can change your eating habits once and for all.

TURN TO GOD

The transformation from food addiction cannot come from dietary boundaries and self-control alone; it must come from God helping you. Turn to the Lord when you want to eat inappropriately. Explore your emotions with him and ask him to stabilize your feelings. Allow him to minister to your heart and mind, and your eating habits will improve. Use your journal to help you know what is triggering your temptations and ask God to help you overcome these specific triggers.

Memorize his Word so you can live by it and recite it. Turn to him when your journey gets tough. Do not count on your self-control as you have in the past; count on him. Hand over control of your eating habits to the Lord. Relinquish the outcome of your lifestyle change to God. Submit your life to him. Live in victory through total reliance on him. If you do, you will be transformed by a renewing of your mind as indicated in Romans 12:2: "Don't copy the behavior and customs of this world, but let God transform you into a new person by changing the way you think. Then you will learn to know God's will for you, which is good and pleasing and perfect." Be patient and trust God for he is faithful.

My sister feels like a new person. Her rosacea disappeared, as well as her excess weight. Her joints no longer ache. Big chores, like house cleaning, don't seem like such a difficult task for her to accomplish anymore. She feels good inside and out because the glorious body God gave her healed through providing it with proper nutrition. As you continue to nourish your body, weak-functioning cells will be replaced by new ones, and your body will work to heal itself of diseases the way the Lord intended.

As a Certified Health and Wellness Coach, I encourage and guide others to regain their health. A client told me her pediatric endocrinologist diagnosed her son as obese and prediabetic. We reviewed the types of food her family ate and developed a plan to cut out unhealthy foods. She resolved to eliminate wheat, milk, and fruit juice from her family's diet. I encouraged her to try to improve their eating habits 80 percent of the time and not worry about what they ate the other 20 percent of the time, since no one can be perfect. If you would like me to assist you on this journey to improve your health as your wellness coach go to SusanUNeal.com/Health-Coaching.

SIX-MONTH SELF-ASSESSMENT

You started this journey with a self-assessment of your physical health. Six months after you start this program, perform another assessment. At that time, record your results here and note the healthy improvements you will have experienced.

Date:

Weight:

Waistline:

Cognitive Assessment Results:

Put a check by the following unhealthy symptoms you still experience.

_____ Fatigue
_____ Foggy brained
_____ Poor memory
_____ Insomnia
_____ Irritability

_____ Mood swings

_____ Anxiety

_____ Depression

_____ Hormonal imbalance

_____ Decreased sex drive

_____ Chronic fatigue, fibromyalgia

_____ Craving sweets and refined carbohydrates or alcohol

_____ Digestive issues: bloating, constipation, diarrhea

_____ Skin and nail infections such as toenail fungus, athlete's foot, and ringworm

_____ Vaginal yeast infections, urinary tract infections

In the space below, write the types of food you ate for the past week. Recalling these foods will test your memory (which should have improved). Note the difference between the foods you just ate and those you recorded in step 1, which are the foods you ate before you began the process of making a lifestyle change.

_____

_____

_____

_____

CONTINUE THE JOURNEY

Understand this is a spiritual battle as well as a physical one. But you can break free from the control of food. God is full of grace and mercy to help you. He is not condemning but loving. Be loving of yourself while you are on this journey to a healthier you, the you God created you to be.

Hebrews 12:1–2 states, "Let us strip off every weight that slows us down, especially the sin that so easily trips us up. And let us run with endurance the race God has set before us. We do this by keeping our eyes on Jesus, the champion who initiates and perfects our faith." I pray you attain the results you desire in obtaining a body that functions well. Be sure to give your body the organic foods God created.

Dear friend, I am praying that all is well with you and that your body is as healthy as I know your soul is.

3 John 2 (TLB)

Blessings, Susan Neal

TAKING STEP 7: IMPROVE YOUR HEALTH

Congratulations on taking these seven steps to get off sugar and carbs and improve your health, life, and future! As you continue on with these lifestyle changes, remember to utilize the following actions steps:

1. Remember the 80/20 percent rule. If you improve your eating 80 percent of the time you will improve your diet and health. However, healing takes time so be patient.

2. Expect to stumble. No one is perfect, but give yourself grace, as God does, when you do mess up and eat poorly.

3. Rely on God. Turn to him and the Bible verses you memorized when you stumble.

4. Document your path to recovery in your journal. How do you look at food? Are you using food to comfort and meet an emotional need, or do you think of food as a necessity to keep your body functioning? Have you journaled about this? Do you turn to food to help

you deal with the challenges of life? If so, food is your stronghold. Learn from your mistakes as you record what occurred, and figure out why so you can prevent these mishaps in the future.

5. Hand over control of your eating habits to the Lord. Relinquish the outcome of your lifestyle change to God. Submit your life to him. Live in victory through total reliance on him.

6. Perform your self-assessment at six months into your journey. Compare this assessment to the first one you took at the beginning of this journey. Note your areas of improvement in your journal and let these victories motivate you to continue to improve and maintain your new healthy lifestyle.

7 Steps to Get Off Sugar and Carbohydrates:

Step 1. Decide to improve your health through proper nutrition.

Step 2. Acquire a support system and knowledge to help make a lifestyle change.

Step 3. Clean out your pantry and refrigerator by removing unhealthy foods and clean out your emotions.

Step 4. Purchase healthy foods and an anti-Candida cleanse.

Step 5. Plan for the start date to begin changing your eating habits.

Step 6. Prepare and eat foods differently than you did before.

Step 7. Improve your health through continuing this new lifestyle never turning back to your old eating habits.

APPENDIX 1: SCRIPTURE VERSES

When you experience temptation, negative emotions, or sinful thoughts regarding your journey to a healthy lifestyle, speak the Word of God out loud and thrust the sword of the Spirit toward the evil forces that might be influencing you. Spoken Bible verses become a double-edged sword to defeat the enemy. State these scripture verses boldly and with authority, believing in their power. This offensive weapon drives the enemy away from you. But first, repent of any sins.

These scripture verses are categorized into various topics you might face in your journey to wholeness. You may find others to add to this list. Seek to memorize as many as you can so you can mentally access them whenever you need to call upon the power of God's Word in your daily battles. To help in memorization, I suggest you write individual verses and their references on an index card to carry with you as you go.

ADDICTION

I can do anything I want to if Christ has not said no, but some of these things aren't good for me. Even if I am allowed to do them, I'll refuse to if I think they might get such a grip on me that I can't easily stop when I want to.

1 Corinthians 6:12 (TLB)

We demolish arguments and every pretension that sets itself up against the knowledge of God, and we take captive every thought to make it obedient to Christ.

2 Corinthians 10:5 (NIV)

Let us strip off every weight that slows us down, especially the sin that so easily trips us up. And let us run with endurance the race God has set before us. We do this by keeping our eyes on Jesus, the champion who initiates and perfects our faith.

Hebrews 12:1–2

Teach me to do your will, for you are my God. May your gracious Spirit lead me forward on a firm footing.

Psalm 143:10

Each time he said, "My grace is all you need. My power works best in weakness." So now I am glad to boast about my weaknesses, so that the power of Christ can work through me.

2 Corinthians 12:9

And let us not get tired of doing what is right, for after a while we will reap a harvest of blessing if we don't get discouraged and give up.

Galatians 6:9 (TLB)

Rather, clothe yourselves with the Lord Jesus Christ, and do not think about how to gratify the desires of the flesh.

Romans 13:14 (NIV)

I have been crucified with Christ and I no longer live, but Christ lives in me. The life I now live in the body, I live by faith in the Son of God, who loved me and gave himself for me.

Galatians 2:20 (NIV)

No discipline seems pleasant at the time, but painful. Later on, however, it produces a harvest of righteousness and peace for those who have been trained by it.

Hebrews 12:11 (NIV)

Therefore, I urge you, brothers and sisters, in view of God's mercy, to offer your bodies as a living sacrifice, holy and pleasing to God—this is your true and proper worship.

Romans 12:1(NIV)

"It is not by force nor by strength, but by my Spirit, says the Lord of Heaven's Armies."

Zechariah 4:6

Well then, shall we keep on sinning so that God can keep on showing us more and more kindness and forgiveness? Of course not! Should we keep on sinning when we don't have to? For sin's power over us was broken when we became Christians and were baptized to become a part of Jesus Christ; through his death the power of your sinful nature was shattered. Your old sin-loving nature was buried with him by baptism when he died; and when God the Father, with glorious power, brought him back to life again, you were given his wonderful new life to enjoy.

Romans 6:1–4 (TLB)

ANGER

And "don't sin by letting anger control you."

Ephesians 4:26

Stop being angry! Turn from your rage! Do not lose your temper—it only leads to harm.

Psalm 37:8

A gentle answer turns away wrath, but a harsh word stirs up anger.

Proverbs 15:1 (NIV)

A hot-tempered person starts fights; a cool-tempered person stops them."

Proverbs 15:18

ANXIETY AND WORRY

"So be strong and courageous! Do not be afraid and do not panic before them. For the LORD your God will personally go ahead of you. He will neither fail you nor abandon you."

Deuteronomy 31:6

"So don't worry about tomorrow, for tomorrow will bring its own worries. Today's trouble is enough for today."

Matthew 6:34

Don't worry about anything; instead, pray about everything. Tell God what you need, and thank him for all he has done. Then you will experience God's peace, which exceeds anything we can understand. His peace will guard your hearts and minds as you live in Christ Jesus.

Philippians 4:6–7

DEPRESSION / DISCOURAGEMENT / DESPAIR

The eyes of the LORD watch over those who do right; his ears are open to their cries for help. But the LORD turns his face against those who do evil; he will erase their memory from the earth. The LORD hears his people when they call to him for help. He rescues them from all their troubles.

Psalm 34:15–17

Why am I discouraged? Why is my heart so sad? I will put my hope in God! I will praise him again—my Savior and my God!

Psalm 42:5–6

He will call on me, and I will answer him; I will be with him in trouble, I will deliver him and honor him. With long life I will satisfy him and show him my salvation.

Psalm 91:15–16 (NIV)

But God, who encourages those who are discouraged, encouraged us by the arrival of Titus.

2 Corinthians 7:6

FEAR

I prayed to the LORD, and he answered me. He freed me from all my fears.

Psalm 34:4

For God has not given us a spirit of fear and timidity, but of power, love, and self-discipline.

2 Timothy 1:7

Be strong and courageous. Do not be afraid or terrified because of them, for the LORD your God goes with you; he will never leave you nor forsake you.

Deuteronomy 31:6 (NIV)

But even if you suffer for doing what is right, God will reward you for it. So don't worry or be afraid of their threats.

1 Peter 3:14

GUILT AND CONDEMNATION

But if we confess our sins to him, he is faithful and just to forgive us our sins and to cleanse us from all wickedness. If we claim we have not sinned, we are calling God a liar and showing that his word has no place in our hearts.

1 John 1:9–10

Who dares accuse us whom God has chosen for his own? No one—for God himself has given us right standing with himself. Who then will condemn us? No one—for Christ Jesus died for us and was raised to life for us, and he is sitting in the place of honor at God's right hand, pleading for us.

Romans 8:33–34

For God made Christ, who never sinned, to be the offering for our sin, so that we could be made right with God through Christ.

2 Corinthians 5:21

HATRED

"So now I am giving you a new commandment: Love each other. Just as I have loved you, you should love each other. Your love for one another will prove to the world that you are my disciples."

John 13:34–35

"But I say, love your enemies! Pray for those who persecute you! In that way, you will be acting as true children of your Father in heaven."

Matthew 5:44–45

INSECURITY

As soon as I pray, you answer me; you encourage me by giving me strength.

Psalm 138:3

Our purpose is to please God, not people. He alone examines the motives of our hearts.

1 Thessalonians 2:4

"Don't be afraid, for I am with you. Don't be discouraged, for I am your God. I will strengthen you and help you. I will hold you up with my victorious right hand."

Isaiah 41:10

For I am convinced that neither death nor life, neither angels nor demons, neither the present nor the future, nor any powers, neither height nor depth, nor anything else in all creation, will be able to separate us from the love of God that is in Christ Jesus our Lord.

Romans 8:38–39 (NIV)

JEALOUSY

I am not saying this because I am in need, for I have learned to be content whatever the circumstances.

Philippians 4:11 (NIV)

And this same God who takes care of me will supply all your needs from his glorious riches, which have been given to us in Christ Jesus.

Philippians 4:19

Yet true godliness with contentment is itself great wealth. After all, we brought nothing with us when we came into the world, and we can't take anything with us when we leave it. So if we have enough food and clothing, let us be content.

1 Timothy 6:6-8

LONELINESS

Turn to me and have mercy, for I am alone and in deep distress.

Psalm 25:16

"And be sure of this—that I am with you always, even to the end of the world."

Matthew 28:20 (TLB)

"And I will be your Father, and you will be my sons and daughters, says the LORD Almighty."

2 Corinthians 6:18

MERCY

Because of the LORD's great love we are not consumed, for his compassions never fail. They are new every morning; great is your faithfulness.

Lamentations 3:22–23 (NIV)

PRAYER

And pray in the Spirit on all occasions with all kinds of prayers and requests. With this in mind, be alert and always keep on praying for all the Lord's people.

Ephesians 6:18 (NIV)

REJECTION

"You didn't choose me. I chose you."

John 15:16

Even before he made the world, God loved us and chose us in Christ to be holy and without fault in his eyes. God decided in advance to adopt us into his own family by bringing us to himself through Jesus Christ."

Ephesians 1:4–6

But despite all this, overwhelming victory is ours through Christ who loved us enough to die for us.

Romans 8:37 (TLB)

REVENGE

Dear friends, never avenge yourselves. Leave that to God, for he has said that he will repay those who deserve it. Don't take the law into your own hands.

Romans 12:19 (TLB)

"I will take revenge; I will pay them back. In due time their feet will slip. Their day disaster will arrive, and their destiny will overtake them."

Deuteronomy 32:35

"The LORD will grant that the enemies who rise up against you will be defeated before you. They will come at you from one direction but flee from you in seven."

Deuteronomy 28:7 (NIV)

SELFISHNESS

Don't think only of yourself. Try to think of the other fellow, too, and what is best for him.

1 Corinthians 10:24 (TLB)

He died for all so that all who live—having received eternal life from him—might live no longer for themselves, to please themselves, but to spend their lives pleasing Christ who died and rose again for them.

2 Corinthians 5:15 (TLB)

SPIRITUAL WARFARE

For I can do everything God asks me to with the help of Christ who gives me the strength and power.

Philippians 4:13 (TLB)

"Look, I have given you authority over all the power of the enemy."

Luke 10:19a

"You, dear children, are from God and have overcome them, because the one who is in you is greater than the one who is in the world."

1 John 4:4 (NIV)

For though we live in the world, we do not wage war as the world does. The weapons we fight with are not the weapons of the world. On the contrary, they have divine power to demolish strongholds. We demolish arguments and every pretension that sets itself up against the knowledge of God, and we take captive every thought to make it obedient to Christ.

2 Corinthians 10:3-5 (NIV)

STRESS

Give all your worries and cares to God, for he cares about you.

1 Peter 5:7

"And besides, what's the use of worrying? What good does it do? Will it add a single day to your life? Of course not! And if worry can't even do such little things as that, what's the use of worrying over bigger things?

"And don't worry about food—what to eat and drink; don't worry at all that God will provide it for you. All mankind scratches for its daily bread, but your heavenly Father knows your needs. He will always give you all you need from day to day if you will make the Kingdom of God your primary concern."

Luke 12:25–26, 29–31 (TLB)

TEMPTATION

Submit yourselves, then, to God. Resist the devil, and he will flee from you.

James 4:7 (NIV)

There he told them, "Pray that you will not give in to temptation."

Luke 22:40

Don't do as the wicked do. Avoid their haunts—turn away, go some-where else.

Proverbs 4:14–15 (TLB)

God is our refuge and strength, an ever-present help in trouble.

Psalm 46:1 (NIV)

For God is working in you, giving you the desire and the power to do what pleases him.

Philippians 2:13

My son, if sinful men entice you, do not give in to them. My son, do not go along with them, do not set foot on their paths."

Proverbs 1:10, 15 (NIV)

"Watch and pray so that you will not fall into temptation. The spirit is willing, but the flesh is weak."

Mark 14:38 (NIV)

Happy is the man who doesn't give in and do wrong when he is tempted, for afterwards he will get as his reward the crown of life that God has promised those who love him.

James 1:12 (TLB)

No temptation has overtaken you except what is common to mankind. And God is faithful; he will not let you be tempted beyond what you can bear. But when you are tempted, he will also provide a way out so that you can endure it.

1 Corinthians 10:13 (NIV)

UNFORGIVENESS

"But when you are praying, first forgive anyone you are holding a grudge against, so that your Father in heaven will forgive your sins, too."

Mark 11:25

Be kind and compassionate to one another, forgiving each other, just as in Christ God forgave you.

Ephesians 4:32 (NIV)

A further reason for forgiveness is to keep from being outsmarted by Satan, for we know what he is trying to do.

2 Corinthians 2:11 (TLB)

APPENDIX 2: CHRISTIAN WEIGHT LOSS AND FOOD ADDICTION PROGRAMS

First Place 4 Health (FirstPlace4Health.com) offers a biblical approach to weight loss through a series of Bible studies. Online groups are available, or you can check to see if one exists in your area.

Take Back Your Temple (TakeBackYourTemple.com) is a Christian online weight loss program whose motto is "Your body for God's glory. We help you take back your house so you can fulfill your God-given purpose."

The Eden Diet: A Biblical and Merciful Anti-Dieting Plan for Weight Loss (TheEdenDiet.com) is a Christian weight-loss program with online support groups.

Thin Within: A Non-Diet Grace Based Approach (ThinWithin.org) is a Christian weight management program that includes online classes and groups.

Barb Raveling Christian weight loss products (Barb Raveling.com) include, a podcast—Taste for Truth: Christian Weight Loss, an app—I Deserve a Donut: and Other Lies That Make You Eat, and a couple of books—*Taste for Truth: A 30 Day Weight Loss Bible Study* and *I Deserve a Donut: And Other Lies that Make You Eat.*

Grace Filled Plate (GraceFilledPlate.com) is a website with an excellent blog which includes having a healthy mindset, recipes, nutrition, and faith.

Victory Steps for Women: Christian Weight Loss & Spiritual Wellness (VictorySteps.net/christian-weight-loss-program.html) is a faith-based health and wellness coaching program, helps women overcome emotional eating, binge eating, and compulsive overeating behaviors.

Weight Loss, God's Way (CathyMorenzie.com/challenge/) is a Christian-based weight loss program that offers a free twenty-one-day challenge.

Three different online food addiction programs include:
OA.org/ (OA is Overeater's Anonymous)
FoodAddicts.org/
FoodAddictsAnonymous.org/

Joining an online support group is another way to share the ups and downs of this journey. Connecting with like-minded individuals who are persevering through the same trials as you helps divide the load. Through these support groups, you can exchange acquired knowledge about your shared journey. In addition, sometimes we need to vent and express our disappointment or success with another person who understands. Life sharing nourishes the emotional side of our well-being.

APPENDIX 3: HEALTHY LIVING JOURNAL

Write the following items in your journal:

1. The time you eat.
2. Why you want to eat. Are you hungry, bored, angry? Is it just "time to eat" or are you with others who are having a meal?
3. If you feel a strong emotion related to this consumption of food, record the emotion.
4. Food you ate and drank, including quantity.
5. How you feel after you ate? Are you satisfied or stuffed?
6. Energy level and clarity of mind after you ate.
7. When waking up in the morning, how do you feel? See if there is a pattern of eating high-sugar-content foods and feeling sluggish the next morning.
8. What are you grateful for today?
9. Prayer requests to God.
10. Exercise—type of activity and length of time.
11. Number of glasses of water you drank and when. Did you drink on an empty stomach?
12. Every time you binge, record: what you ate, why you ate it,

what triggered you to eat it, and what you might do the next time you are tempted.

As you write this information, recognize any patterns between your emotions and food consumption. Did you eat because you were hungry? If no, why?

APPENDIX 4: RECIPES

The following recipes will help you keep sugar and refined carbohydrates out of your diet and still enjoy delicious meals made with whole, natural foods. The recipes are divided into breakfast, snacks/desserts, dips, vegetables/side dishes, entrees, and bread.

BREAKFAST

Granny Sue's Granola
    8 cups organic oats
    1 cup almonds
    1 cup pecans
    1 cup walnuts
    ½ cup sunflower seeds
    $^1/_3$ cup sesame seeds
    1/3 cup pumpkin seeds
    ¾ cup coconut or olive oil
    ½–2/3 cup of honey
    Combine all ingredients. Pour into two large greased baking pans. Bake at 325 degrees for 18–20 minutes; take out and stir. Cook for

another 18–20 minutes, stir and add the following ingredients: 1–2 cups of dried fruit—berries, dates, apricots, raisins, or craisins.

Cook for 10 more minutes. Store granola in two-quart mason jars. Put one on the kitchen counter and the other in the refrigerator. Makes two quarts.

Banana Pancakes

1 smashed banana (lower in sugar if green)
1 egg
½ cup almond flour
1 tablespoon coconut oil
¼ teaspoon baking soda

Combine all ingredients. Cook just like a pancake, but make the cakes small, so they are easier to flip.

Strawberry/Almond Coffee Cake

Preheat oven to 350 degrees and spray an 8X8 pan with olive oil.
2½ cups almond flour
½ teaspoon baking soda
¼ teaspoon salt
¼ cup melted coconut oil
1 tablespoon honey or maple syrup
1 teaspoon baking stevia
1 teaspoon vanilla

Combine all ingredients with a mixer.

Fold 2 cups diced strawberries into the mix.

Put in the pan and add the following topping.

Topping

½ cup almond flour
3 tablespoons softened coconut oil
1 tablespoon honey or maple syrup
1 teaspoon baking stevia
½–1 cup sliced almonds

Combine topping ingredients (except nuts) with a pastry cutter.

Add nuts and sprinkle mixture on top of the coffee cake. Bake for 25–30 minutes until a toothpick comes out clean.

Apple Quinoa Breakfast Muffins

Preheat oven to 375 degrees. Spray a muffin pan with olive oil.

1 cup cooked quinoa

½ cup applesauce

1 mashed banana (lower in sugar if green)

½ cup almond or coconut milk

1 tablespoon honey or maple syrup

2 teaspoons baking stevia

1 teaspoon vanilla

1 teaspoon cinnamon

2½ cups orgainic oats

1 chopped apple

Mix all ingredients. Pour ingredients into muffin pan. Bake for 20–25 minutes.

Chia Parfait

4 tablespoons chia seeds

1 cup almond or coconut milk

½ teaspoon cinnamon

1 teaspoon vanilla

$1/_8$ teaspoon baking stevia

1 cup of fruit of your choice (berries, banana—lower in sugar if green)

½ cup of organic oats

½ cup slivered almonds (or another nut)

Mix the first five ingredients and put in the refrigerator overnight.

In the morning layer the chia mixture with oats, nuts, and fruit in parfait glasses. Top with fresh fruit. (Makes 4 servings.)

Hash Brown Cups

Preheat oven to 350 degrees. Spray muffin pan with olive oil.

1 bag shredded hash browns

3 chopped green onions
½ teaspoon salt
¼ teaspoon pepper
2 tablespoons olive oil
Combine all ingredients. Spoon into muffin pan. Bake for 60–75 minutes. Makes 12 muffins.

Banana Quinoa Oatmeal
1 cup of quinoa cooked in 2 cups of water (about 4 cups cooked)
2 smashed slightly green bananas (lower in sugar if green)
¾ cup chopped walnuts
1 teaspoon cinnamon
1 teaspoon vanilla
1 tablespoon honey or 1 teaspoon of stevia
¾ cup almond or coconut milk
Combine ingredients on stovetop and warm.

Banana Egg Pancakes
1 smashed banana (lower in sugar if green)
2 eggs
$^1/_8$ teaspoon cinnamon
Mix ingredients together and pour small-sized pancakes in a hot skillet so they flip easily. These delicious pancakes need no syrup because the banana is sweet. (Makes one serving.)

Apple Oatmeal Cups
Preheat oven to 350 degrees and spray muffin pan with olive oil.
2 cups organic oats
1 teaspoon baking soda
$^1/_8$ teaspoon salt
½ teaspoon cinnamon
1 cup almond or coconut milk
1 egg
1 mashed banana (lower in sugar if green)
1 diced apple

Mix all ingredients. Pour into a muffin pan and bake for 20–25 minutes.

SNACKS/DESSERTS

Dehydrated Fruit

A food dehydrator is a terrific investment when beginning to change to a healthier style of eating. Simply cut your fruit into similar sized slices. Place on dehydrator trays and turn on for the length of time indicated by your dehydrator's instructions. If the fruit is in different sizes, the small pieces will get overdone, and the large pieces will not be completely dried. Store dried fruit in mason jars. I give specific instructions on how to dehydrate foods in my YouTube video at Youtube.com/c/SusanNealScriptureYoga.

Coconut Macaroon Cookies

    3 egg whites
    ¼ teaspoon salt
    1 teaspoon vanilla
    1–2 teaspoon stevia
    1 tablespoon monk fruit sugar
    1½ cups unsweetened, shredded coconut

Whip the egg whites and vanilla until peaks form. Fold the rest of the ingredients into the whipped egg whites. Let mixture stand for 5 minutes. Bake for 10–15 minutes on a greased cookie sheet at 350 degrees until the macaroons are lightly brown.

Frozen Berries

Either pick or purchase your berries (organic is best). Rinse with water and drain in a colander. Place berries on an ungreased cookie sheet. Make sure the berries do not touch. Place in freezer several hours until frozen. Place frozen berries in mason jars and put in the freezer. Since the berries are frozen individually, you can take as much or as little out of the jar as you need when making your fruit smoothie. My youngest daughter loved to crunch on frozen blueberries.

Berry Smoothie

1 cup coconut or almond milk

1 cup frozen berries

1 teaspoon coconut oil

Stevia to sweeten

1 cup ice

Protein smoothie: add ½ cup of nuts (almond, pecan, walnut) or 2 tablespoons of almond butter.

Green smoothie: add ½ cup of spinach or kale.

Dark Chocolate–Covered Nuts, Seeds, and Currants

Melt 1–2 bars of dark chocolate (at least 70 percent cocoa), which is healthy and low in sugar. Add a mixture of nuts, seeds, and currants until coated. Drop by tablespoons onto a sheet of wax paper. As the mixture cools, the nut clusters will harden.

Granny Sue's Cranberry Relish

1 large package of raspberry-cranberry Jello

Replace ¾ cup of sugar (from the Jello package's directions) with appropriate measurement of powdered stevia, monk fruit sugar, or half and half mixture.

Prepare the Jello as directed, using the sugar substitute, and place in refrigerator.

Meanwhile, chop the following ingredients by hand or in food processor:

2 cups apples

2 cups celery

2 cups lightly roasted pecans

12-oz package of cranberries

Mix these four ingredients into the Jello and refrigerate until firm.

Dark Chocolate Chip Pecan Cookies

3 cups of almond flour (could substitute 1 cup with coconut flour)

¼ teaspoon salt

1 teaspoon baking soda

¼ cup of coconut or olive oil

1 teaspoon of stevia for baking

¼ cup of maple syrup

1 egg

1 teaspoon vanilla

½ cup dark chocolate chips (more than 70 percent cocoa)

½ cup pecans, almonds, or walnuts (optional)

Combine dry ingredients. In a separate bowl, mix oil, stevia, syrup, eggs, and vanilla with a hand mixer. Slowly add dry ingredients. Mix by hand when adding chocolate chips and nuts. Bake at 375 degrees for 15 minutes.

Almond Butter

Bake almonds for 15 minutes at 325 degrees on an ungreased cookie sheet.

Let almonds cool and place them in a food processor.

Blend on high for about 7–10 minutes. Stop and stir the mixture about every minute.

If you like crunchy nut butter, take a few tablespoons of nuts out of the food processor after blending it for about 30 seconds. I set five tablespoons aside for a one-pint mixture.

Store in the refrigerator.

Almond Flour

Bake almonds for 15 minutes at 325 degrees on an ungreased cookie sheet.

Let almonds cool and place them in a food processor.

Blend on high for about 2–3 minutes until it is the consistency of uncooked grits.

Store in a pint jar in the refrigerator or freezer. Use it just like you would white flour.

Trail Mix

2 cups almonds

2 cups walnuts

2 cups pecans

1 cup sunflower seeds

½ cup sesame seeds

¾ cup raisins

¾ cup craisins

Mix all ingredients together and store in the refrigerator.

Organic Popcorn

2 tablespoons coconut oil

¼–$^1/_3$ cup organic popcorn kernels (1 serving)

Cook oil and popcorn on high in a pan with a lid on the stove top.

Toppings: ½–1 tablespoon butter, 1 tablespoon olive oil, kelp, dulse (seaweed), sea salt

DIPS

Guacamole

5–6 smashed avocados

½ cup diced cherry tomatoes

2 tablespoons cilantro

2 tablespoons olive oil

2 tablespoons red wine vinegar

½ cup chopped purple onion or scallion

2 cloves minced garlic (use fresh garlic, not from a jar)

1 tablespoon lime juice

Mix all ingredients together. Leave the avocado pits in the dip for better storage.

Hummus

1 cup sesame seeds

1 clove of garlic

2 tablespoons olive oil

Bake sesame seeds at 350 degrees for 20 minutes. Put roasted seeds in food processer with 1 garlic clove and 2 tablespoons of oil. This is tahini. Set aside.

4 cups dried garbanzo beans

> 3 lemons juiced
> ½ cup lemon zest
> ½ teaspoon salt
> ½ teaspoon cumin

Soak garbanzo beans in water overnight. Pour out water. Cook garbanzo beans in water that is one inch over the top of the beans for 40 minutes or until tender. Cool and drain but set aside 1 cup of the water. Blend the beans and rest of ingredients in the food processor. If needed, add some of the water you set aside until the consistency of the mixture is creamy. Add the tahini and blend.

VEGETABLES/SIDE DISHES

Barb's Asian Slaw

> 1 cabbage head, shredded
> 4 chopped green onions
> ½ cup slivered or sliced almonds

Dressing

> ½ cup olive oil
> ¼ cup tamari or soy sauce
> 1 tablespoon honey or maple syrup
> 1 tablespoon baking stevia

Heat up dressing ingredients in a saucepan on the stove until thoroughly mixed.

Mix all ingredients when you are ready to serve.

Blueberry Cantaloupe Avocado Salad

> 1 diced cantaloupe
> 2–3 chopped avocados

1 package of blueberries
¼ cup olive oil
$^1/_8$ cup balsamic vinegar
Mix all ingredients.

Beet Salad (from Israel)

2–3 fresh, raw beets grated or shredded in food processor
3 tablespoons olive oil
2 tablespoons balsamic vinegar
¼ teaspoon salt
$^1/_3$ teaspoon cumin
Dash stevia powder or liquid
Dash pepper
Mix all ingredients together for the best raw beet salad.

Broccoli Salad

1 head broccoli, chopped
2–3 slices of fried bacon, crumbled
1 diced green onion
½ cup raisins or craisins
½–1 cup of chopped pecans
¾ cup sunflower seeds
½ cup of pomegranate

Dressing
1 cup organic mayonnaise
¼ cup baking stevia
2 teaspoons white vinegar
Mix all ingredients together. Mix dressing and fold into salad.

Rosemary Garlic Potatoes

Preheat oven to 425 degrees.
5 red new potatoes, chopped
¼ cup olive oil
2–3 cloves of minced garlic

1 tablespoon rosemary

Stir all ingredients together in a bowl. Pour onto a baking sheet and bake for 30 minutes.

Sweet and Sour Cabbage

1 tablespoon honey or maple syrup

1 teaspoon baking stevia

2 tablespoons water

1 tablespoon olive oil

¼ teaspoon caraway seeds

¼ teaspoon salt

$1/_8$ teaspoon pepper

2 cups chopped red cabbage

1 diced apple

Cook all ingredients in a covered saucepan on the stove for 15 minutes.

Barley and Lentil Salad

1 head romaine lettuce

¾ cup cooked barley

2 cups cooked lentils

1 diced carrot

¼ chopped red onion

¼ cup olives

½ chopped cucumber

3 tablespoons olive oil

2 tablespoons fresh lemon juice

Mix all ingredients together. Add kosher salt and black pepper to taste.

ENTREES

Homemade Chicken Broth

1 tablespoon olive oil

1 chopped onion

    2 chopped stalks celery

    2 chopped carrots

    1 whole chicken

    2+ quarts of water

    1 tablespoon salt

    ½ teaspoon pepper

    1 teaspoon fresh sage

Sauté vegetables in oil. Add chicken and water and simmer for 2+ hours until the chicken falls off the bone. Keep adding water as needed. Remove the chicken carcass from the broth, place on a platter, and let it cool. Pull chicken off the carcass and put it into the broth. Pour broth mixture into pint and quart mason jars. Be sure to add meat to each jar. Leave one full inch of space from the top of the jar or it will crack when it freezes as liquids expand. Place jars in freezer for up to a year. Take out and use whenever you make a soup.

Homemade Vegetable Broth

    1 tablespoon olive oil

    1 chopped onion

    2 chopped stalks celery

    2 chopped carrots

    1 head bok choy

    6 cups or 1 package fresh spinach

    2+ quarts of water

    1 tablespoon salt

    ½ teaspoon pepper

    1 teaspoon fresh sage

Sauté vegetables in oil. Add water and simmer for 1 hour. Keep adding water as needed. Pour broth mixture into pint and quart mason jars. Leave one full inch of space from the top of the jar or it will crack when it freezes as liquids expand. Place jars in freezer for up to a year. Take out and use whenever you make a soup.

Fish Stew

    1 tablespoon olive oil

1 chopped onion or leek
2 chopped stalks celery
2 chopped carrots
1 clove minced garlic
1 tablespoon parsley
1 bay leaf
1 clove
$^1/_8$ teaspoon kelp or dulse (seaweed)
¼ teaspoon salt
Fish—leftover, cooked, diced
2–3 cups chicken or vegetable broth
Add all of ingredients and simmer on the stove for 20 minutes.

Quinoa with Vegetables

2 cups water
1 cup dried quinoa
Assorted fresh vegetables
Cook quinoa in water.
Sauté an assortment of vegetables in olive oil. Different vegetable combinations include:

- sautéed scallions, mushrooms, and spinach along with sunflower and pumpkin seeds;

- sautéed onion, bell peppers, and kale with a fresh avocado on top;

- sautéed bok choy, snow peas, and carrots with cashews and sesame seeds.

Either serve vegetables on top of quinoa or combine.

Black Bean Soup

1 pound dry black beans (soak in water overnight and drain water)
1 tablespoon olive oil

2 cups chopped onion or 1 leek

1 cup chopped carrots

4 cloves minced garlic

2 teaspoons cumin

¼ teaspoon red pepper flakes

4 cups chicken broth

4 cups water

¼ teaspoon thyme

2 chopped tomatoes or 1 (14 oz) can tomatoes

1½ teaspoon salt

Optional: add bacon or ham to flavor

Chopped green onions to garnish

Sauté vegetables in oil. Add rest of ingredients and cook on stovetop on medium-low heat for 1 hour.

Richard's Best Chicken

2 tablespoons olive oil

8 chicken thighs

6 cloves garlic

1 jar artichoke hearts, drained

¾ cup chicken broth

3 fresh squeezed oranges

1 sliced Meyer lemon

¼ cup capers

½ cup olives

In a cast-iron skillet, fry chicken on each side in oil until skin is golden and crispy. Remove from skillet. Sauté garlic and artichokes for a few minutes, add chicken (skin up). Pour in rest of ingredients and bring to a boil. Place skillet with all ingredients uncovered in a 350-degree oven for 30 minutes.

White Bean and Cabbage Soup

1 tablespoon olive oil

4 chopped carrots

4 chopped stalks of celery or 1 chopped bok choy

1 chopped onion

2 cloves minced garlic

1 chopped cabbage head

½ lb northern beans soaked in water overnight (drained)

6 cups chicken broth

3 cups water

Sauté vegetables in oil. Add rest of ingredients and cook on medium-low heat for 30 minutes.

Brooke's Chili

2 lb organic ground beef

1 diced onion

3 cloves minced garlic

6 diced tomatoes

1 jar tomato sauce

1 tablespoon salt

1 cup water

1 cup kidney beans soaked in water overnight (drained)

1 cup pinto beans soaked in water overnight (drained)

2 tablespoons chili powder

1 tablespoon cumin

1 tablespoon honey or maple syrup

1 teaspoon baking stevia

1 teaspoon pepper

In a large pot, brown the ground beef and drain the grease. Add the onion and garlic and cook until translucent. Add rest of ingredients and simmer for 1 hour.

Lentil Soup

2 tablespoons olive oil

2 chopped onions

1 chopped red pepper

1 chopped carrot

2 cloves minced garlic

½ teaspoon cumin

¾ teaspoon thyme

1 bay leaf

8 cups chicken broth

2 chopped tomatoes

½ pound dried lentils (1¼ cup)

Optional: add bacon or ham to flavor

1 teaspoon salt

¼ teaspoon pepper

Handful of spinach

Sauté vegetables in oil. Add rest of ingredients (except spinach and spices). Cover and cook on low for 2 hours. Add spinach and spices.

White Chicken Chili

1 tablespoon olive oil

1 pound of chicken strips cut into pieces

2 teaspoons cumin

½ teaspoon oregano

½ teaspoon salt

½ teaspoon pepper

1 chopped onion

1 chopped red bell pepper

4 cloves minced garlic

4 cups chicken broth

2 cups northern beans soaked in water overnight (drained)

Sauté chicken and spices in oil and remove from pan. Sauté onion and red pepper. Add rest of ingredients including chicken and cook on medium-low heat for 15 minutes.

Mixed Vegetable Soup

1 tablespoon olive oil

1 chopped leek

1 chopped bok choy

4 chopped carrots

2 cloves minced garlic

1 chopped zucchini

2 chopped tomatoes

1 cup garbanzo beans soaked in water overnight (drained)

5 chopped potatoes

8 cups broth

1 teaspoon basil

½ cup amaranth

Sauté first four ingredients, add garlic for last minute. Add rest of ingredients and simmer on the stove for 25 minutes.

Potato Soup

2 tablespoons olive oil

1 diced onion

4 minced cloves garlic

1 teaspoon thyme

1 bay leaf

4 diced red potatoes

6 cups water

1 sliced leek

3 diced celery stalks

2 teaspoons salt

¼ teaspoon pepper

Sauté onion, garlic, thyme, and bay leaf in oil until translucent. Add rest of ingredients and simmer for about 20 minutes.

BREAD

Granny Sue's Corn Pone

Preheat oven to 440 degrees and spray a cookie sheet with olive oil.

¼ teaspoon salt

1 cup oatmeal

1 cup organic cornmeal

¼ cup sesame seeds

¼ cup sunflower seeds

¼ cup pumpkin seeds

1 cup hot water

Combine all ingredients and stir.

Pour mixture onto a greased cookie sheet and shape like large oval cookies about ½ inch thick. Bake for 35 minutes.

Kim's Gluten Free, Dairy Free, Whole Grain Bread[1]

3 large eggs lightly beaten

1 teaspoon apple cider vinegar

¼ cup oil of choice (canola, olive, corn, coconut, grapeseed, etc.)

1¹/₃ cup milk of choice—unsweetened (rice, hemp, almond, cow) warmed to about body temperature

1 tablespoon +1 teaspoon honey

3 tablespoons brown sugar

½ cup millet, sorghum, quinoa, amaranth, or buckwheat flour (choose one)

½ cup second choice of flour: millet, sorghum, quinoa, amaranth, or buckwheat flour (choose one)

1 cup multigrain rice flour, brown rice flour, or (my favorite) teff flour

½ cup tapioca flour

½ cup cornstarch (potato starch works too)

3 teaspoons xanthan gum

1½ teaspoons salt

2¼ teaspoons dry active yeast

optional add ins:

flax seeds

sesame seeds

sunflower seeds

add in a total of about a ¼ cup

Combine first six ingredients in bread maker pan. Sift next seven ingredients and then add on top of liquid ingredients. Toss in your add ins. Make a little well in the dry ingredients and add the yeast in the hole. Start the bread maker on the gluten-free bread setting. Gluten-free bread needs less time as there is no need for additional punch downs like with wheat bread.

APPENDIX 5: HEALTHY EATING GUIDELINES

Low-carbohydrate, anti-inflammatory dietary guidelines include:

- About 50 percent of food items are fresh organic vegetables.
- Eat one fresh, raw serving of low-glycemic fruit per day. Low-glycemic fruits include green apples, berries, cherries, pears, plums, and grapefruit.
- Do not always eat cooked foods. Eat a couple of servings of raw vegetables every day. Have a salad for lunch with either nuts or meat. When eating out, order a salad or coleslaw as sides, since both are raw.
- Another 25 percent of your daily food intake should come from an animal or vegetable protein such as beans, nuts, and lean meats. Fish is exceptionally nutritious. Try to eat it once a week.
- A variety of different nuts and seeds are excellent sources of protein, minerals, and essential fatty acids.
- Avoid sugar, flour, rice, pasta, and bread. Instead, eat more fruits, vegetables, and low-glycemic grains such as quinoa and pearled barley.
- Do not eat sugary cereals. Instead, eat oatmeal, fruit, or

granola. Be careful, as the sugar content of granola may be high. My favorite granola recipe appears in appendix 4.

- Try not to eat anything containing more than 10 grams of sugar in one serving, or 24 grams for a woman or 36 grams for a man per day.
- Eat nontraditional grains such as quinoa, amaranth, pearled barley, wild rice, and oats.
- Eat cultured foods such as kimchi, sauerkraut, and cultured plain Greek yogurt since they contain natural probiotics. Add one to two tablespoons of these foods to a meal twice a week or eat the yogurt as a snack. Personally, I take a probiotic capsule every day.
- Replace undesirable ingredients with whole foods. *The Daniel Plan Cookbook* by Rick Warren provides a chart titled Foods and Ingredients to Avoid and suggests replacements. A few recommendations from this book include:
- Replace sugary snacks with nuts, nut butter, dark chocolate, and plain Greek yogurt with berries.
- Replace condiments and sauces containing MSG or high-fructose corn syrup with spices, vinegar, and herbs.
- Replace table salt with kosher or sea salt.
- Replace fried foods with baked foods.

APPENDIX 6: SEVEN-DAY EATING PLAN

Day 1 (Start on Wednesday)

1. Consume Water

Drink up to two cups of coffee or tea per day, but no more. The only other beverage you should drink is filtered water. I use a filter on my refrigerator water dispenser and a water filter on a pitcher. Before breakfast drink two glasses of water, two before lunch, two midafternoon, and two more before dinner. Do not drink during meals and do not drink anything after dinner. Drink up to ten minutes before eating.

2. Take a Probiotic

Begin taking a probiotic every day. I usually buy several probiotics from a health food store with at least ten different strains of beneficial bacteria, and I take a different one each day to vary the flora in my gastrointestinal system. I store my probiotics in the refrigerator door. After I take a probiotic, I move the bottle to a different shelf, so I can keep track of the one I took last.

3. Stop Eating High-Sugar Foods

Stop eating anything containing greater than 10 grams of sugar per serving, or 24 grams for a woman or 36 grams for a man per day. Check labels for the number of grams of sugar per serving size.

Day 2

1. Eliminate Wheat

Do not eat anything containing wheat. No more bagels, toast, pancakes, biscuits, pasta, pretzels, crackers, cookies, cake, or pie. Eliminating wheat is like going off a drug. Be aware that you may experience the following symptoms for a few days: irritability, foggy brain, and fatigue. You might even feel fluish. However, within a week your symptoms will subside. After this, never eat wheat or more than 10 grams of sugar in one serving again, or your addiction will start all over again. (Ugh.)

Day 3

1. Eliminate Processed Foods

Do not eat processed foods from boxes and bags.

2. Implement Healthy Eating Guidelines

Make 50 percent of your food fresh and raw. Follow the Healthy Eating Guidelines provided in appendix 5.

Days 4 and 5 (Saturday and Sunday)

Continue to implement all the steps listed on day one through three as you proceed.

1. Rest

Focus on you. Rest, read, pray, and ask God to help you to succeed.

2. Use the Sword of the Spirit

Now is the time to fight the thief Jesus spoke of in John 10:10, for Satan wants you to fail: "The thief's purpose is to steal, kill and destroy. My purpose is to give life in all its fullness" (John 10:10 TLB).

Fight the thief with the sword of the Spirit—the Word of God. Write verses on index cards or put them on the notes app on your smartphone. Use verses that will remind you of the help God provides in any struggles you may be facing at this point, such as Philippians 4:13: "For I can do everything through Christ, who gives me strength." Every time you get the urge to go back to your old eating habits, speak the verse out loud to cut the demonic influence out of your life. Our spiritual nature needs to be addressed as well as our physical.

Day 6

1. Start the Anti-Candida Cleanse

Now let's kill the bug in your gut—Candida. Today, start the anti-Candida cleanse you purchased in step 4. If you are not ready to begin this step because you are still experiencing symptoms of withdrawal (headache, exhaustion, irritability, mental fogginess, fluish symptoms), wait a few days until you feel better. Read the instructions on the cleanse package for how to administer it. Initially, I recommend taking the cleanse every other day for the first week to minimize lethargy and headaches. You will feel awful if the dead Candida is not quickly expelled from your colon. To avoid becoming constipated, drink plenty of water. During the second week, begin taking the Candida cleanse every day as recommended.

Prevent a headache by increasing the fiber in your diet through a fiber supplement (which usually comes with your Candida cleanse), water, and raw fruits and vegetables. The first three days you are on the cleanse, you may not feel well, but after a week you will begin to feel better than you have in a long time. You are just about to get the life back Jesus wants you to experience—one that is abundant and full.

Day 7

1. Get Up and Exercise

If you are still feeling the symptoms of withdrawal, be gentle with yourself by performing a simple form of exercise such as walking or yoga. It doesn't matter what type of exercise you do just as long as you do it. Walking, jumping rope, lifting weights, or taking a group fitness class like Pilates or water aerobics are a few examples of exercise. After you begin feeling better, try to exercise for twenty minutes three times a week. Record the exercise you perform in the *Healthy Living Journal* or the journal that you set up in step 2.

Mindfulness exercises such as yoga and meditation train a person to pay attention to cravings without reacting to them. The idea is to ride out the wave of intense desire. As a person becomes more mindful she notices why she wants to indulge. Meditation quiets the part of the brain that can lead to a loop of obsession. Check out my website at ChristianYoga.com.

Day 8 and Beyond

You are well on your way to changing your lifestyle, but more than that you will change your life for the better. Your health, mood, and energy level will improve. Each week you will lose weight, and the body God gave you will heal itself of many ailments. As your body heals the disease processes, you will be able to reduce or eliminate medications because you will no longer suffer from the maladies these medications were treating. However, before stopping any prescription medication be sure to consult with your physician. Improvement in your vitality will allow you to experience activities you were not able to be involved in before. Overall your well-being and emotional countenance will become revitalized. You are in the process of getting your life back, the one that God wants you to enjoy to its fullest.

APPENDIX 7: HOW TO BECOME A CHRISTIAN AND DISCIPLE OF JESUS CHRIST

Accepting Jesus as your Savior

Salvation begins when we recognize our sinfulness and ask God to forgive us. We accept that Jesus Christ humbled himself in obedience to God by dying on a cross to pay for our sins. Sin is simply to miss the mark, to live our lives by our own selfish desires instead of following God's ways.

Since Jesus never sinned, he was an acceptable sacrifice to pay the debt (eternal damnation) for our sins. Once we accept Jesus' gift and ask him to come into our hearts, we are filled with the Holy Spirit. Accepting Jesus places the helmet of salvation on our heads. Our Savior's Spirit within us gives us the ability to come before God and receive his grace and mercy to help us in our times of need.

Accepting Jesus as your savior is simple. All you need to do is pray. In this prayer ask God to forgive you for your sins and tell him that you will turn away from those sins. Ask Jesus to come into your heart and lead your life. At that moment you receive the Holy Spirit.

When we accept Christ as our Savior, God adopts us as his children and loves us unconditionally like a parent. Nothing can take his love away from us. Since we are his children, we can access his power by faith and apply it to any area in our lives.

Becoming a Disciple of Jesus Christ

We become righteous when we ask God to forgive us of our sins and accept Jesus Christ as our Lord and Savior; at that moment God replaces our sin with our Savior's righteousness—since he never sinned. To maintain this right standing, we must accept God's moral standards as our values. Living our life in obedience to those values is part of becoming a disciple of Jesus Christ.

We become Jesus' disciple when we submit our lives to him and allow him to lead us. How do we let Jesus lead our lives? Through following his Word and responding to the prompting of the Holy Spirit inside of us. We should pay attention to the gentle nudging the Spirit gives us and pray throughout the day. Remain in contact with Jesus spiritually through silently talking to him and asking for his help and guidance as you need it. He wants to be a part of your life.

It is important to spend time with God, maybe through reading a devotion or a Bible verse as well as spending meditative time in God's presence. Ask him to lead you and he will. Search for him, and you will find him. Jeremiah 29:13 (NIV) "You will seek me and find me when you seek me with all your heart." So start seeking.

Through salvation, we received the Holy Spirit. Receiving God's Spirit compares to a seed which needs soil, sunlight, water, and fertilizer to grow. As the seed grows so does our faith. The following four habits can help us to stand firm in our faith:

1. Studying and memorizing scripture verses
2. Spending time with the Lord
3. Fellowship with other Christians
4. Submitting control of our lives to Jesus

These practices will make us spiritually strong and wise.

APPENDIX 8: FIVE-STEP BINDING THE STRONG MAN PLAN

1. Name what controls you.

Name the thing controlling you—food addiction, anxiety, eating disorder, depression, etc.—whatever it may be, and declare (out loud) Jesus Christ is your Lord in its place![5]

Stand up to the evil spirit who brought bondage into your life by saying, "Evil spirit, you won't lord over me nor entice me through (insert your addiction) anymore. Jesus is my Lord!" A person obtains spiritual power and authority through Christ. Declare that the spiritual powers of darkness will not have lordship over your life. They will not rule you, govern your behavior, capture your thought life, nor lead you into temptation and sin because "the one who is in you is greater than the one who is in the world" (1 John 4:4 NIV).

"For when Satan, strong and fully armed, guards his palace, it is safe—until someone stronger and better armed attacks and overcomes him and strips him of his weapons and carries off his belongings." Luke 11:21–22 (TLB)

Get ready, for *you are capable of evicting the addiction strong man in your life*. If you accepted Jesus as your Lord and Savior (see appendix 7 to find out how), the Holy Spirit lives within you and the Spirit is stronger than Satan. Day after day, declare out loud that Jesus reigns as the Lord of your life—not your addiction.

2. Submit yourself completely to God.

"Submit yourself to God, resist the devil and he will flee from you." James 4:7 (NIV)

There is a secret to resisting the devil—you must first submit yourself to God. How in the world do you do that? In my experience, you no longer do your will but God's will by submitting your life to him. For me, it was not without a fight.

If you are a food addict, after binging, ask God to forgive you and help you not to binge the next time. Record your experience in your journal. Once you ask for forgiveness, God chooses not to remember your sins, as indicated in Hebrews 8:12: "And I will be merciful to them in their wrongdoings, and I will remember their sins no more" (TLB). Don't fret over a stumble. Get up and try again using this Five-Step Binding the Strong Man Plan.

3. Use the name of Jesus.

Jesus told his disciples, "Look, I have given you authority over all the power of the enemy" (Luke 10:19). If you are a disciple of Jesus (see appendix 7 to find out how) you can accept the authority he gave you.

In the book of Acts, the apostles healed and worked miracles in the name of Jesus. Use Jesus's name as Peter did in Acts 3:6: "in the name of Jesus Christ of Nazareth, walk" (TLB). Using the name of Jesus is key to binding the strong man because then you operate under Jesus's authority.

Picture a person tied in ropes. That's the way a spiritual strong man afflicts his victim. However, if you declare Jesus is Lord over your life, not the strong man (addiction), and use Jesus's name, you are under his authority. Then the ropes, tied around you by the evil spirit, break. Eventually, the spiritual ropes loosen and fall off. Next, comes the moment to take action by tying the strong man through binding him with the Word of God.

4. Use the Word of God.

"For when Satan, strong and fully armed, guards his palace, it is safe—until someone stronger and better armed attacks and overcomes him and strips him of his weapons and carries off his belongings." Luke 11:21–22 TLB

The Holy Spirit inside of you is stronger than Satan and his demons. By using the name of Jesus, you are not only under his authority but you can speak with his authority. You are much better armed than Satan. Now is the time to stand up to him, strip him of his weapons, and kick him out of your life through the Word of God! Say to the strong man, "In the name of Jesus, you won't oppress me anymore. I bind your power in the name of Jesus and by the Word of God."

Search the Bible for a verse that is the opposite of your addiction. A whole selection of verses is provided in appendix 1. Use the specific scripture you chose to bind the strong man every time he tempts you. Write this verse on an index card and memorize it.

Luke 11:22 states the strong man was stripped of his weapons and his belongings were carried off. Matthew 12:29 asserts when Satan was bound his demons could be cast out. After you tie up the strong man with the Word of God—ignore him. He will try to hobble after you because he doesn't give up easily. If he did, he wouldn't be a strong man. Remember, the next time you are tempted, you're facing a critical moment. When you give him (the spirit of addiction) your attention by drinking, eating sugary foods, worrying—whatever addiction it was—you are, in effect, untying the strong man.

5. Praise God and practice gratitude.

When you praise God and thank him for his blessings, the strong man won't hang around. Don't be satisfied with binding the strong man and walking away—punish him.

Fill your mind, heart, and body with the Spirit of God by putting the right things in your spirit. Listen to praise music; read the Bible and pray; memorize scripture; attend church, Sunday school, or a Bible study. Also, start doing more to help others. Performing acts of service and helping others fills your heart with honorable feelings and humility. Every day, write in your journal about all you can praise God for and thank him.

Beat the strong man by declaring Bible verses out loud. Stomp him into the ground by singing praises to God. The devil can't stand to be around someone who worships the Lord.

Become God's warrior by using his mighty unseen weapons. Paul advises, "It is true that I am an ordinary, weak human being, but I don't use human plans and methods to win my battles. I use God's mighty weapons, not those made by men, to knock down the devil's strongholds" (2 Corinthians 10:3–4 TLB). Get ready to knock out and tie up the strong man of addiction in your life. You are God's mighty conqueror!

APPENDIX 9: CURB THE SWEET TOOTH

When the craving for sugar arises, I eat one of these nutritious snacks:

- Slice a green apple, which is low in sugar, and add almond or cashew butter to each slice. It tastes sweet; conversely, the almond butter is high in protein. Both the apple and nut butter provide fiber and fill me up.
- Melt 70-percent dark chocolate in a pan on the stove and add different types of nuts until well coated with the chocolate. Place mounds of nut clusters on wax paper. After an hour they harden. Keep in an airtight container on the counter or refrigerator for a week. Nuts contain fiber and are filling.
- Sparingly eat one date along with seven pecan halves. Dates are high in natural sugar, so you only need a smidgen to attain the sweetness. Don't eat too many dates, which are high in sugar, but instead fill up on the pecans, which are high in protein.
- I grow fruit trees in my yard, so from June through December I pick fresh blueberries, apples, grapes, pears, and

oriental persimmons. I eat one serving of fruit each day either for breakfast or as an afternoon snack.

- Curb sweet cravings by adding a teaspoon of raw, unfiltered, unpasteurized apple cider vinegar in a cup of water with a couple of drops of stevia.

APPENDIX 10: FOOD ADDICTION BATTLE STRATEGIES

1. Record pertinent information listed in appendix 3 in your journal.
2. Find a specific Bible verse to oppose your food issue and write it on an index card. Keep it with you until you memorize it. Speak the verse out loud every time you feel the urge to eat unhealthy foods.
3. Ask a friend to be your accountability and prayer partner.
4. Join a Christian weight loss program or an online food addiction program.
5. Determine food triggers and eliminate them.
6. Implement the Five Steps to Binding the Strong Man Plan:
7. Name the thing controlling you—your food addiction, anxiety, eating disorder, depression, etc.—whatever it may be, and declare (out loud) Jesus Christ is your Lord in its place!
8. Submit yourself completely to God.
9. Bind the strong man (evil spirit of addiction) with the name of Jesus.
10. Use the Word of God to bind the strong man.
11. Punish the strong man by praising God.

Do you have an accountability/prayer partner, yet? Acquiring a support system is integral to successfully make this lifestyle change. Have you joined a Christian weight loss program or one of the online food addiction programs? A list of these programs is provided in appendix 2. If you need to, reread step 2 about how to create your support system.

When you eat any unhealthy food, be sure to journal afterward—every single time. Figure out what you told yourself that validated why it was okay to eat the item. Then go through the Five Steps to Binding the Strong Man Plan (appendix 8). If you journal and implement this five-step plan every time you binge, you will experience success. Retraining your mind is like disciplining a child; consistency is vital to conformity.

NOTES

Step 1

1. William Davis MD, *Wheat Belly* (New York: Rodale Inc., 2011), 8–9, 48–49.
2. Fiona MacDonald, "Watch: This is How Sugar Affects Your Brain," *Science Alert*, November 3, 2015, https://www.sciencealert.com/watch-this-is-how-sugar-affects-your-brain.
3. Rick Warren, Daniel Amen MD, and Mark Hyman MD, *The Daniel Plan: 40 Days to a Healthier Life* (Grand Rapids: Zondervan, 2013), 106–7.
4. Donna Gates, *The Body Ecology Diet* (New York: Hay House, Inc., 2010), 3.
5. Fran Smith, "The Addicted Brain," *National Geographic*, September 2017, 36–37, 42–43.

Step 2

1. Erin Schumaker, "Surgeon General Vivek Murthy:

Addiction is a Chronic Brain Disease, Not a Moral Failing," *Huffington Post,* November 17, 2016.

2. Deane Alban, "How to Increase Dopamine Naturally," Be Brain Fit, Bebrainfit.com/increase-dopamine/.

3. Smith, "Addicted Brain," 36–37, 42–43.

4. Ibid., 36.

5. Ibid., 36–37.

6. "Candida Yeast Infection, Leaky Gut, Irritable Bowel and Food Allergies," National Candida Center, https://www.nationalcandidacenter.com/Leaky-Gut-and-Candida-Yeast-Infection-s/1823.htm.

7. Davis, *Wheat Belly,* 24.

8. Hetty C. van den Broeck, Hein C. de Jong, Elma M. J. Salentin, Liesbeth Dekking, Dirk Bosch, Rob J. Hamer, Ludovicus J. W. J. Gilissen, Ingrid M. van der Meer, and Marinus J. M. Smulders, *"Prescence of celiac disease epitopes in modern and old hexaploid wheat varieties: wheat breeding my have contributed to increased prevalence of celiac disease,"* *Theoretical and Applied Genetics* 121(8), (November 2010): 1527–39, https://www.ncbi.nlm.nih.gov/pmc/articles/PMC2963738/.

9. Ibid.

10. "Candida Yeast Infection, Leaky Gut, Irritable Bowel and Food Allergies."

11. Davis, *Wheat Belly,* 60–63.

12. John Brennan, "What is Roundup Ready Corn," Sciencing, April 25, 2017, https://sciencing.com/roundup-ready-corn-6762437.html.

13. Rebecca Boyle, "How to Genetically Modify a Seed, Step By Step," *Popular Science,* January 24, 2011.

14. Gates, *Body Ecology Diet,* 59–63.

15. Mark Water, *Scripture Memory Made Easy* (Peabody: Hendrickson Publishers, 1999), 9–11.

16. Davis, *Wheat Belly,* 8.

Step 3

1. Smith, "Addicted Brain," 37, 43–44.
2. Davis, *Wheat Belly*, 25–26.
3. Smith, "Addicted Brain," 50.
4. Tom McKay, "What Happens to Your Brain on Sugar: Explained by Science," Mic.com, April 21, 2014, https://mic.com/articles/88015/what-happens-to-your-brain-on-sugar-explained-by-science-.rAKas1ERY.
5. John Brennan, "What is Roundup Ready Corn," Sciencing, April 25, 2017, https://sciencing.com/roundup-ready-corn-6762437.html.
6. Alexandra Sifferlin, "Artificial Sweeteners are Linked to Weight Gain—Not Weight Loss," Time, July 17, 2017, http://time.com/4859012/artificial-sweeteners-weight-loss/.
7. Susan Scutti, "Dangerous Effects of Artificial Sweeteners on Your Health," Medical Daily, July 10, 2013, http://www.medicaldaily.com/4-dangerous-effects-artificial-sweeteners-your-health-247543.
8. Stacy Simon, "World Health Organization Says Processed Meat Causes Cancer," *American Cancer Society*, October 26, 2015, https://www.cancer.org/latest-news/world-health-organization-says-processed-meat-causes-cancer.html.
9. Kris Gunnars, "Why is Coconut Oil Good for You? A Healthy Oil for Cooking," *Health Line*, May 26, 2017, https://www.healthline.com/nutrition/why-is-coconut-oil-good-for-you - section4.
10. Jennifer Hartle, Ana Navas-Acien, Robert Lawrence, "The consumption of canned food and beverages and urinary Bishpenol A concentrations in NHANES 2003–2008," *Environmental Research* Volume 150, (October 2016): 375–76, Sciencedirect.com/science/article/pii/S0013935116302407.
11. "U.S. Food and Drug Administration," "Bishpenol A (BPA):

Use in Food Contact Application" (November 2014),
www.fda.gov/newsevents/publichealthfocus/ucm064437.

12. Tom Valentine, "The Proven Dangers of Microwaves,"
Nexus Volume 2, #25 (April-May 1995),
http://www.mercola.com/article/microwave/hazards2.htm.

13. "What's in Your Pantry?" by Tana Amen BSN, RN and Dr.
Daniel Amen, YouTube, https://www.youtube.com/watch?
v=VqoWO0-RSAI.

Step 4

1. Keri Gardner, "How Acids Affect Calcium in the Teeth &
Bones," *LiveStrong*, August 14, 2017.

2. James Colquhoun, "The Truth About Calcium and
Osteoporosis," *Food Matters*, November 24, 2009,
http://www.foodmatters.com/article/the-truth-about-
calcium-and-osteoporosis.

3. Rick Warren, Daniel Amen MD, and Mark Hyman MD, *The
Daniel Plan Cookbook* (Grand Rapids: Zondervan, 2014),
16–17.

4. Brenda Davy, "Clinical Trial Confirms effectiveness of
Simple Appetite Control Method," *American Chemical
Society*, August 23, 2010, http://www.acs.org.

5. Alexa Fleckenstein, MD, "The Top Foods Inflaming Your
Body," *Rodale Wellness*, November 11, 2014.

6. Donna Gates, *Body Ecology Diet*, 3–8.

7. Perlmutter, *Grain Brain*, 224.

Step 5

1. Darren Warburton, Crystal Nicol, and Shannon Bredin,
"Health Benefits of Physical Activity: The Evidence," *Canada
Medical Association Journal* 174, (March 14, 2006): 801–9.

2. Miriam Reiner, Christina Niermann, Darko Jekauc, and
Alexander Woll, "Long-term Health Benefits of Physical

Activity—A Systematic Review of Longitudinal Studies,"
BioMed Central Public Health, September 8, 2013.
3. Smith, "Addicted Brain," 51.
4. "Bible Commentary," Adam Clarke Commentary,
   https://www.studylight.org/commentaries/acc/matthew-
   12.html.
5. Larry Lea, *The Weapons of Your Warfare: Equipping Yourself to
   Defeat the Enemy* (Reading: Cox and Wyman, Ltd. 1990),
   126, 182.

Step 7

1. James Allen, *As a Man Thinketh* (Orig. pub. 1903; London:
   Value Classic Reprints, 2017).
2. Smith, "Addicted Brain," 36–37.

Appendix 4

1. "Kim's Gluten Free, Dairy Free, Whole Grain Bread," Gluten
   Free Real Food, https://gfrealfood.com/2009/06/10/kims-
   gluten-free-dairy-free-whole-grain-bread/.

CHRISTIAN STUDY GUIDE FOR 7 STEPS TO GET OFF SUGAR AND CARBOHYDRATES

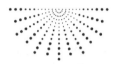

HEALTHY EATING FOR HEALTHY LIVING WITH GOD'S FOOD

Editor: Janis Whipple

Cover Design: Angie Alaya

Printed in the United States of America

ISBN: 978-0-997-76367-6

I would like to dedicate this book to my Bible study groups:

Home Group
Cara, Dru, Judy, Gemell, Karen, Kimberly, Krista, Lauren, Margie, Mo,
Paige, Pam A., Pam P., Pat, Sue, Susan, Suzy, Tanya, Terri, Tess, Tracey

Living Truth Church Group
Anna, Cheryl, Christiana, Dawn, Dianne, Evie, Jeanene, Jen, Jenny, Jessica,
Julie, Kathryn, Karen J., Karen L., Kristi, Megin, Melinda, Navannah, Pat,
Ruthann, Sarah, Shannon, Shirley, Stephanie, Tangee, Tara, Teresa, Theresa

May God bless your endeavor to improve your health.

Dear friend, I hope all is well with you and that you are as healthy in body as
you are strong in spirit.
3 John 2

DISCLAIMER

Medical Disclaimer: This book offers health and nutritional information, which is for educational purposes only. The information provided in this book is designed to help individuals make informed decisions about their health; it is intended to supplement, not replace, the professional medical advice, diagnosis, or treatment of health conditions from a trained medical professional. Please consult your physician or healthcare provider before beginning or changing any health or eating habits to make sure that it is appropriate for you. If you have any concerns or questions about your health, you should always ask a physician or other healthcare provider. Please do not disregard, avoid, or delay obtaining medical or health-related advice from your healthcare professional because of something you may have read in this book. The author and publisher assume no responsibility for any injury that may result from changing your health or eating habits.

Disclaimer and Terms of Use: Every effort has been made to ensure the information in this book is accurate and complete. However, the author and publisher do not warrant the accuracy or completeness of the material, text, and graphics contained in this book. The author and publisher do not hold any responsibility for

errors, omissions, or contrary interpretation of the subject matter contained herein. This book is presented for motivational, educational, and informational purposes only. This book is sold with the understanding that the author and publisher are not engaged in rendering medical, legal, or other professional advice or services. Neither the publisher nor the author shall be liable for damages arising herein.

PREFACE

Dear Reader,

I want to help you recover your health and ideal weight by teaching you which foods are beneficial and which ones make you sick. In this study we will mobilize God's power to evoke lifestyle changes you may struggle to implement on your own. You can change your future by changing the types of food you eat.

Will you join me on a journey to obtain the abundant life God wants you to live? I hope you will!

Blessings,

Susan U. Neal

INTRODUCTION

When I was fifty I lost my health. I had no idea how precious it was until it was gone. I laid in bed, utterly exhausted, unable to function normally. It all began when an abscessed tooth poisoned my body. Over the next year, I developed ten medical diagnoses, endured two surgeries, and gained an unhealthy amount of weight. The doctors did all they could, but I still was not well.

As a registered nurse with a master's degree in health science, I used my medical knowledge and the Bible to recover my health and weight. Taking a biblical approach to master my palate, I eliminated the foods I knew I should not eat. I want to share what I learned, so you can achieve the extraordinary life God wants you to experience.

I created this Christian study guide for three purposes:

1. To provide an opportunity for individuals to implement the steps in *7 Steps to Get Off Sugar and Carbohydrates* in a small group. Accountability improves a person's chance for success.
2. To apply biblical wisdom to different situations that may hold a person back from making necessary lifestyle changes. This approach will help you grow spiritually and

teach you how to access God's mighty power to make the changes you need.

3. So other individuals can benefit from the knowledge I gained when I cured myself of my illnesses.

I hope you take this journey to recover your health and achieve all the blessings the Lord has in store for you.

HOW TO USE THIS STUDY

The purpose of this Christian study guide is to reinforce the principles from the book *7 Steps to Get Off Sugar and Carbohydrates*. Therefore, you will need a copy of the book as you work through this guide. In addition, tracking your physical, emotional, and spiritual health in a journal is the best way to gain freedom from any food issues you may experience. You can create your own journal to use with this guide, or purchase the *Healthy Living Journal*.

A corresponding video series titled, 7 Steps to Reclaim Your Health and Optimal Weight is available at SusanUNeal.com/courses/7-steps-to-get-off-sugar-and-carbs-course. This course includes an introductory video and syllabus which explain how to proceed with the study. Seven videos, one for each step, are part of the course along with handouts.

This Christian study guide is intended for use in a group setting, along with individual daily lessons (five per week). However, the steps in this guide can be implemented on your own. In the group setting you will:

1. Discuss what you learned and incorporated into your life over the past week.

2. Read the corresponding chapter in *7 Steps to Get Off Sugar and Carbohydrates.*
3. Answer the questions in the study guide.

You can't change your lifestyle overnight. An accountability group can propel you to achieve your healthy living goals. Each week you will be challenged to make new changes. At the end of the seven weeks, your life will be transformed from the inside out!

To provide additional support, I would like to invite you to join my closed Facebook group: 7 Steps to Get Off Sugar and Carbohydrates.

Leader's Guide

A Leader's Guide is provided at the end of the book. Leader instructions are provided in *italics* throughout the book.

GROUP GUIDELINES

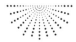

During this study we will ask participants to share openly with each other. The following guidelines will establish a healthy group experience.

- Make a commitment together that the group will be a place of safety and confidence. No one will share what they hear, so all information will be kept confidential.
- Commit to support each other through encouragement and prayer.
- Resolve to grow spiritually, physically, mentally, and emotionally.
- Make group attendance a priority. Notify the leader if you will be absent or late.

PART I

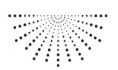

[PART]

SESSION 1: DECIDE TO IMPROVE YOUR HEALTH

Our society faces an epidemic because over half of Americans live with a chronic illness and forty percent suffer from obesity.[1] What caused this epidemic? I believe it is the foodlike substances that manufacturers entice us to eat. Instead, we need to eat the foods our Creator designed for humans.

God gave you a glorious body that can heal itself if you provide it with the proper nutrition he intended. However, you need to find out what foods are beneficial versus harmful. Through gaining knowledge and using the Lord's spiritual arsenal, this Christian study guide will help you reclaim the abundant life God wants you to live.

When you implement the steps in this study, you will improve the way you feel and look and increase your energy and clarity of mind. You will lose weight naturally without going on a fad diet or buying prepared meals and supplements. These results can be achieved by merely changing the types of food you eat. Through commitment, self-examination, and the Lord's help, you will improve your health.

You may think the Bible doesn't say anything about eating carbohydrates and sugar. True, but our bodies are the temple of the Holy Spirit; therefore, our Creator expects us to take care of our bodies. When you make healthy eating choices, you nurture and support your body so that it can last a lifetime. If you are healthy, you can fulfill the unique purpose God has planned for you. Also you will enjoy being a godly influence in the lives of those you love for a longer period of time, so you can help them reach their God-given potential.

Despite God's desire for his children to enjoy long, abundant lives on earth, the lifespan of Americans is declining.[2] I believe a major contributing factor to the decline is the consumption of too much sugar and refined carbohydrates. From my experience, it is difficult to wean oneself off of these addictive substances, therefore, I created the following seven-step plan:

7 Steps to Get Off Sugar and Carbohydrates

1. **Decide** to improve your health through proper nutrition. Biblically we will address addiction, generational bondage, and abuse. To help us on our journey, we will learn the importance of the sword of the Spirit.
2. **Acquire** a support system and knowledge to help make a lifestyle change. We are stronger when Christian friends support us during this transition. Humility versus pride is addressed by studying King Saul's mistakes. To obtain a balanced ego, we need our identity to originate from Christ.
3. **Clean out** the pantry and refrigerator by removing unhealthy foods, and clean out your emotions. Emotional and stress eating may relate to unhealed emotional wounds and unforgiveness. We discuss how to heal the wounds from the past.
4. **Purchase** healthy foods plus an anti-Candida cleanse. Sin is compared to yeast (Candida). Also we look at Daniel's resolve in Babylon when he refused to eat the king's food. Like Daniel, we can stand firm by changing our mind-set.
5. **Plan** a start date and begin to change your eating habits. This lesson teaches five steps to obtain freedom from food

addiction. We learn how to use the Lord's power as we wear the armor of God.

6. **Prepare** and eat foods differently than you did before. We review and ensure implementation of all the action steps provided in steps 1–7.

7. **Improve** your health through continuing this new lifestyle, never turning back to your old eating habits. Celebrate your achievements, victories, and transformation.

In your study group, you will learn how to utilize God's divine power to evoke lifelong changes rather than rely on self-control. This book differs from other healthy living books because we learn to equip ourselves with spiritual weapons to attain victory.

This plan is not a diet but a lifestyle change. However, the guidelines are not so stringent that you feel like you have a noose around your neck. You apply God's wisdom along with accurate knowledge about today's food.

For session one, read the introduction and first chapter, titled Step 1: Decide to Improve Your Health, in *7 Steps to Get Off Sugar and Carbohydrates*. You might take turns reading it aloud with each member reading a paragraph. When you get to the section titled, "Make Your Commitment" on page 11, stop reading and finish your session by filling out the information below. Whatever portion of the chapter you are not able to finish should be assigned as homework.

Prepare for Commitment

You may be experiencing a health crisis and need to make a change. This book will walk you through the process to regain your health, so you can feel energetic again and begin to live the purposeful life God intended for you.

To begin this journey, evaluate your current health situation by answering the questions below. The answers will help you set goals for improvement to restore wholeness to your life.

Health Problems

Many health problems can keep you from an abundant life. Place a checkmark by each symptom you experience:

_____ Overweight

_____ Lack of energy

_____ Joint pain

_____ Ulcer

_____ Diabetes

_____ Allergies

_____ Sinus issues

_____ Take medication

_____ High blood pressure

_____ Autoimmune disease

_____ Bloating, gas, indigestion

_____ Constipation, diarrhea, or other gastrointestinal (GI) problem

_____ Skin problem—eczema, rosacea, rash

_____ Other _____

Share with the group which symptoms are most problematic for you.

_____

Do you struggle with any of the following issues related to your physical health? Check all that apply:

_____ Self-consciousness of weight/appearance

_____ Can't keep up with family members
_____ Clothes don't fit and need to buy more
_____ Guilt when you overeat
_____ Low self-esteem
_____ Moodiness
_____ Depression
_____ Other _____

This assessment gives you a picture of your health. The more items you identified with above, the more your body has been negatively affected by harmful foods. As you change the types of food you eat, your health will improve. A reassessment will be provided in session 7, so you can compare the lists to see if your symptoms decreased.

Food Knowledge and Mental Ammunition

Have you ever found yourself eating something you thought was nutritious, only to find out later that it wasn't? In our society it is difficult to navigate diet trends. In the 1980s, low-fat diets were the trend; now the ketogenic diet is popular. These eating methods seem to be the exact opposite. Which one is best?

Lack of knowledge is a key reason people fall into the trap of unintentionally eating the wrong types of food. When people gain knowledge, they recognize that their previous beliefs were false, and it becomes easier to overcome unhealthy eating habits.

Another reason some people struggle to eat healthy foods is their bodies betray their mental commitment. It may not be just a matter of self-control; you may have a food addiction or overgrowth of Candida in the GI tract that causes you to overeat. We need to recognize how addictions affect us physically, so we can be prepared with the mental ammunition needed to stay strong. Through this study you will learn how to stop the cravings and unwanted symptoms associated with a diet loaded with carbs, and how to arm your mind and spirit with the tools to win this battle.

If you did not watch this five-minute video, please watch it now: Ted-Ed video "How Does Sugar Affect the Brain?" by the neuroscientist Nicole Avena Ph.D., Sciencealert.com/watch-this-is-how-sugar-affects-your-brain.[3]

Are you surprised that sugar is an addictive substance like drugs? Discuss this issue with the group.

_____

Science shows that a biochemical addiction occurs in the brain.[4] The body gets used to the dopamine and craves even more foods high in sugar and refined carbohydrates (processed foods). The person feels an initial "high" from the dopamine release, but soon the body experiences a "crash." When the sugar rush subsides, they feel tired, foggy brained, and downright ill. Then they regret what they ate. When a person gets stuck in this addiction cycle of euphoria and regret, it ultimately leads to health issues and excess weight.

Unfortunately, processed foods promote diseases such as diabetes, hypertension, obesity, and some types of autoimmune diseases. You may feel the adverse effects in your body and are seeking a solution. I pray you will implement the steps in this guide, because they will help you.

The difficulty in this journey for a Christian is that when we are sick we tend to focus on ourselves instead of serving God. Doctor visits, laboratory tests, medications and their side effects, pain, etc. may consume a person's life if he or she is ill. Are you fed up with the state of your health or weight?

This book will help you break the unhealthy eating cycle. In turn, your health and weight will improve. *When we are healthy, we can serve God better.*

Are you ready to reclaim your health? Then *make the decision* to stop eating sugar and refined carbohydrates. Deciding is the first step of the seven-step plan. I challenge you to take the first step—decide to improve your health.

Baseline Assessment

Before changing your eating habits, obtain a baseline of your current condition. Weigh yourself and measure your waistline. This information is private and not to be shared with other members of your group. (*Leader: this section can be performed in your group or on their own.*)

Date:

Weight:

Waistline:

Symptom Checklist

Put a check by the unhealthy symptoms you experience:

_____ Fatigue

_____ Anxiety

_____ Insomnia

_____ Irritability

_____ Depression

_____ Mood swings

_____ Poor memory

_____ Food allergies

_____ Foggy brained

_____ Decreased sex drive

_____ Hormonal imbalance

_____ Chronic fatigue, fibromyalgia

_____ Vaginal yeast infections, urinary tract infections

_____ Craving sweets and refined carbohydrates or alcohol

_____ Digestive issues (bloating, constipation, diarrhea) or disorders

_____ Skin and nail infections such as toenail fungus, athlete's foot, and ringworm

Share with the group which symptoms are most problematic for you.

_____

Dietary Assessment

Recall what foods you ate last week. How difficult is it for you to remember what you ate? Difficulties may indicate memory problems. Studies are beginning to show a connection between sugar and dementia and Alzheimer's disease.[5] We will discuss this further in the study.

Record the foods you ate last week. Please circle the foods that are a refined carbohydrate, or contain wheat or sugar.

_____

_____

. . .

Do wheat, sugar, or processed foods comprise a large part of your diet? These are the types of food you want to avoid.

Accountability/Prayer Partner

Obtaining a support system helps address the emotional and spiritual aspects of your physical transformation. As Ecclesiastes 4:12 tells us, "Though one may be overpowered, two can defend themselves. A cord of three strands is not quickly broken" (NIV). This scripture provides biblical insight about gaining strength through a support system, so you can change your eating habits and break the cycle of unhealthy eating.

Having a friend for accountability who you can call when temptation arises is crucial to your success. It is powerful when a friend speaks the truth in love. Pray with your friend and ask her to pray for you. Prayer is one of our offensive, spiritual weapons (Ephesians 6:18).

Who could be your ally during this lifestyle change? It might be someone in your study group, a good friend, or spouse. Write down the name of someone who you will ask to help you during this journey to improve your health.

. . .

Implement the biblical wisdom found in Ecclesiastes 4:12 and obtain a prayer/accountability partner. When you have made a commitment together, sign your names together here:

(Your Name)

(Accountability Partner's Name)

In addition to obtaining an accountability partner, I would like to invite you to join my closed Facebook group: 7 Steps to Get Off Sugar and Carbohydrates.

Journal

During the next seven weeks, commit to spend a few minutes each day recording what you ate and drank and how your body reacted to these foods. Food issues you didn't know you had will become apparent. Create a journal of your own using the guidelines provided in appendix 3 of *7 Steps to Get Off Sugar and Carbohydrates* or purchase the corresponding *Healthy Living Journal*.

Through recording the information included in a journal, you will begin to solve a puzzle, one you couldn't figure out on your own. You will discover how to make your body feel good again. Each day's entry helps you record water intake, exercise, energy level, daily food intake, and corresponding moods. Through journaling you will learn more about yourself, discover negative health patterns, draw closer to God, and experience better health.

. . .

Personal Goals

What type of improvements would you like to see as a result of this study?

_____

_____

Would you like to share with the group what you hope to achieve?

Conclusion

You are about to embark on a journey to improve the stewardship of your body. You only have one body, and it needs to last a lifetime. During the next week, please complete days 1–5. When you return for session 2, you will discuss this material.

For those who want to jump right in with dietary changes, try not to eat anything with more than 10 grams of sugar at one sitting and stop eating refined carbohydrates (such as snack items you find in boxes and bags). The American Heart Association recommends you limit your calories from sugar to no more than half of your total calories, which is a lot. For most women in the US that should be no more than 24 grams of sugar or 100 calories per day. For men it is 36 grams of sugar or 150 calories from sugar per day.

Healthy snack and menu ideas are listed in the Menu Planning section in Step 6: Prepare and Eat Foods Differently in *7 Steps to Get Off Sugar and Carbohydrates*.

As a group, decide whether you want to read the second chapter of *7 Steps to Get Off Sugar and Carbohydrates*, Step 2: Acquire a Support System and Knowledge, on your own or during session 2.

If you prefer to receive more guidance, a corresponding video series titled, 7 Steps to Reclaim Your Health and Optimal Weight is available at SusanUNeal.com/courses/7-steps-to-get-off-sugar-and-carbs-course. This course includes an introductory video and syllabus which explain how to proceed with the study. Seven videos, one for each step, are part of the course along with handouts.

DAY 1: FOOD ADDICTION TRAP

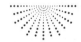

Food addiction is quite prevalent in our society today. It is a biochemical disorder that cannot be controlled through self-control. An addiction causes a person to repeat the same type of behavior despite life-damaging consequences. That is why we need to learn to use God's spiritual weapons.

Read the first four pages of the second chapter, Step 2: Acquire a Support System and Knowledge in *7 Steps to Get Off Sugar and Carbohydrates*. Were you surprised to learn that at some point, an overconsumption of sugar and refined carbohydrates rewires the brain's neural pathways and causes a person to become addicted? No wonder so many people have fallen into the *food addiction trap*. Entitlement leads to indulging, which leads to addiction. It is a slippery slope once you take your first bite of that addictive food. Down the slope you fall as you consume the whole package—which you never intended to do.

In your main small group session, you learned about food addiction in the Ted-Ed video, "How Does Sugar Affect the Brain?": Sciencealert.com/watch-this-is-how-sugar-affects-your-brain. Since dopamine releases when you eat sugar, it makes a person feel so good that it leads to an addiction.

. . .

Do you think you have a food addiction? Journal your thoughts here:

_____

_____

If you think you have a food addiction, do not feel shame. It is not your fault. Your body has fallen prey to the accumulative effects of the standard American diet.

Take a food addiction test at one of these online food addiction programs:

oa.org/ (OA is Overeater's Anonymous)
foodaddicts.org/
foodaddictsanonymous.org/

Record the results of your food addiction test: _____

The foods we eat also affect our brain function. A diet high in sugar is linked to dementia and Alzheimer's. Scientific studies revealed a low-glycemic, low-carbohydrate diet helps prevent and improve these prevalent, devastating diseases.[6]

If you are concerned about your brain health, you can take an online cognitive test to determine the health of your brain. For a free test go to to ElderGuru.com and click on the Sage Alzheimer's Exam on the right lower panel. Record your results here: _____

DAY 2: KING SOLOMON'S ADDICTION

An addiction is a compulsion to engage in an activity whether the person truly wants to or not. Many addictions ruin a person's life. Today we will look at a biblical character whose royal lineage was ruined due to an addiction. Similarly, a food addiction can cause diseases that decrease a person's lifespan, and it may reduce their quality of life too.

King Solomon was a wise king who had an addiction. First Kings 11:3 states, "He had 700 wives of royal birth and 300 three concubines. And in fact, they did turn his heart away from the LORD." Can you imagine having seven hundred royal weddings? He ruled Israel for forty years; that means he got married an average of every three weeks! And this does not include the time it would take to fit three hundred concubines into his life.

Weren't seven hundred wives enough for him? Why did he acquire three hundred concubines too? That would mean that he had a new woman every ten days during his forty-year reign as king. That is a lot of women.

Why do you think King Solomon did this?

. . .

_____

Was it the excitement from having sex? Dopamine, a feel-good neuro-hormone, releases when we enjoy sex, eat foods high in sugar, take opiate drugs, smoke cigarettes, drink alcohol, cuddle with our kids, or pet a dog.[7] Addictions can be related to physical things like food, sex, and drugs, or emotional connections like TV/media, pornography, gaming, and gambling. Some addictions are to things that are good in themselves. For instance, exercise is beneficial, but excessive exercise can become an addiction.

As a person becomes addicted, the dopamine rush rewires the brain to desire more of whatever causes its release. Therefore, when an addict sees the item he desires, dopamine releases and causes his focus to narrow.[8] He can think only about the item of addiction so he can experience the euphoria it brings.

What do you think King Solomon was addicted to? _____

It must have been a time-consuming job to find King Solomon a new wife or concubine every ten days. We know from scripture that Solomon married many foreign women: "Now King Solomon loved many foreign women. Besides Pharaoh's daughter, he married women from Moab, Ammon, Edom, Sidon, and from among the Hittites" (1 Kings 11:1, NLT).

However, God strictly forbid the Israelites to marry non-Israelites: "The LORD had clearly instructed the people of Israel, 'You must not marry them, because they will turn your hearts to their gods.' Yet Solomon insisted on loving them anyway" (1 Kings 11:2, NLT).

. . .

Why would this wise king marry women from other nations when the Lord forbid it?

Did Solomon have a habit that he couldn't stop? Do you have an overeating problem that you can't stop? Addiction is a compulsive repetition of an activity despite life-damaging consequences. For King Solomon, the results were monumental because his foreign wives turned his heart away from God: "As Solomon grew old, his wives turned his heart after other gods, and his heart was not fully devoted to the LORD his God, as the heart of David his father had been. He followed Ashtoreth the goddess of the Sidonians, and Molek the detestable god of the Ammonites" (1 Kings 11:4–5, NIV).

If you have a food addiction, what have the consequences been for you?

Ultimately, Solomon's addiction to women resulted in him worshiping other gods. Because of his idolatry, God took the kingdom of Israel away from his descendants:

The LORD was very angry with Solomon, for his heart had turned away from the LORD, the God of Israel, who had appeared to him twice. He had warned Solomon specifically about worshiping other gods, but Solomon did not listen to the LORD's command. So now the LORD said to him, "Since you have not kept my covenant and have disobeyed my decrees, I will surely tear the kingdom away from you and give it to one of your servants."

1 Kings 11:9–11 (NLT)

King Solomon had wealth, wisdom, and a great kingdom. Yet his addiction led him to disobey God.

Do you have something you are addicted to? What is it?

_____

If you want to be released from this addiction, ask the Lord to help you by writing your prayer below.

_____

_____

_____

_____

Step 5 in *7 Steps to Get Off Sugar and Carbohydrates* provides a spiritual plan to release you from bondage through addiction.

DAY 3: GENERATIONAL BONDAGE

Have you ever noticed that some bad habits or addictions seem to run in families? Alcoholism, smoking, racism, and abuse, to name a few. The skeletons in the closet (sins of the past) play out all over again in another generation. Consequently, an inclination toward a specific type of sin can be passed on from generation to generation because the child learns the behavioral or attitudinal problem. That is why parents and grandparents should be careful about what they sow in the lives of their descendants.

Poor eating habits are also passed down. If a parent typically prepares frozen casserole dishes and processed food, she teaches her children to eat this type of food as well. Gaining knowledge about healthy foods is one way to change this unhealthy eating pattern.

Today we will look at Solomon's dad, King David. Did David commit a sexual sin that influenced his son? Yes, he had sex with Bathsheba, who was married to Uriah. Bathsheba conceived a child, so David had Uriah killed in battle.

Ultimately, David asked God for forgiveness, but he still faced the consequences of his sins, as we read in 2 Samuel 12:9–14:

"Why, then, have you despised the word of the LORD and done this horrible deed? For you have murdered Uriah the Hittite with the sword of the Ammonites and stolen his wife. From this time on, your family will live by the sword because you have despised me by taking Uriah's wife to be your own. This is what the LORD says: Because of what you have done, I will cause your own household to rebel against you. I will give your wives to another man before your very eyes, and he will go to bed with them in public view. You did it secretly, but I will make this happen to you openly in the sight of all Israel."

Then David confessed to Nathan, "I have sinned against the LORD." Nathan replied, "Yes, but the LORD has forgiven you, and you won't die for this sin. Nevertheless, because you have shown utter contempt for the word of the LORD by doing this, your child will die."

Though David repented, and God forgave him for committing adultery and murdering Uriah, he still received the penalties of his sins, and those consequences affected his family. The child that David and Bathsheba initially conceived died, and David's family would "live by the sword" and "rebel against him."

David also had numerous wives:

These are the sons of David who were born in Hebron:

The oldest was Amnon, whose mother was Ahinoam from Jezreel.

The second was Daniel, whose mother was Abigail from Carmel.

The third was Absalom, whose mother was Maacah, the daughter of Talmai, king of Geshur.

The fourth was Adonijah, whose mother was Haggith.

The fifth was Shephatiah, whose mother was Abital.

The sixth was Ithream, whose mother was Eglah, David's wife.

These six sons were born to David in Hebron, where he reigned seven and a half years.

Then David reigned another thirty-three years in Jerusalem. The sons born to David in Jerusalem included Shammua, Shobab, Nathan, and Solomon. Their mother was Bathsheba, the daughter of Ammiel. David also had nine other sons: Ibhar, Elishua, Elpelet, Nogah, Nepheg, Japhia, Elishama, Eliada, and Eliphelet. These were the sons of David, not including his sons born to his concubines. Their sister was named Tamar.

1 Chronicles 3:1–9

How many sons and wives did David have?

_____

How long did he reign? _____

King David's pattern of having multiple wives certainly didn't help his complicated family life. I bet the stepbrother/stepmother arrangement was confusing for Solomon as he grew up. I expect the depth of the relationship David sowed with his nineteen sons was shallow. Solomon may not have known that fathers and sons could have a deep connection, as this may not have been demonstrated to him. I wonder if Solomon was close to any of his siblings, or were they all vying for the throne, which put them in competition with one another?

We can see from King David's generational legacy that an inclination toward a particular type of behavior can be passed down from generation to generation—as modeled by the parent or guardian. This is particularly true of addictive behaviors (such as a food addiction), and physical and sexual abuse. If a parent deals with their problems by consuming excess amounts of food or alcohol, a child may learn to do this as well. If a parent abuses a child, the child (when grown up) may be more likely to harm his or her own child or grandchild.

Abuse can hold a person in bondage. It held me captive for over two decades. Sometimes these chains seem natural because the person grew up with them and doesn't know that there is something different. However, the Lord wants to break the chains of bondage and rebuild the lives of those who were abused. He also wants to change the patterns for that family to break the generational cycle.

Jesus said:

"The Spirit of the Lord is on me, because he has anointed me to proclaim good news to the poor. He has sent me to proclaim freedom for the prisoners and recovery of sight for the blind, to set the oppressed free,"

Luke 4:18 (NIV)

Jesus wants to release you from your bondage. Emotional wounds can effect a person's health. We need healing from the inside out. When we heal from devastating wrongs from our past, it helps us restore our physical bodies too. It could also cure a dysfunctional eating behavior caused by those wounds.

Have you suffered from an abusive situation? If yes, how long did it last, and what affect has it had on different areas of your life?

_____

_____

. . .

I did. I remember the day I exposed my ugly past to my Women of the Word Bible study group. My heart resonated in my chest as I forced the words out of my mouth. Time stood still. Dragging the abuse out of the closet took all my willpower. I hadn't told a soul in twenty-five years, not even my husband.

However, after those words escaped from my heart, I felt relief. The sky did not fall; lightning did not strike. In fact, it seemed anticlimatic. The secret enslaved me for decades. Why hadn't I told anyone? Because I was petrified of what they would think of me, so I never did, until our Bible study group did a Beth Moore study.

During those weeks I realized I was a victim, especially when we examined the verse Matthew 18:6: "If anyone causes one of these little ones—those who believe in me—to stumble, it would be better for them to have a large millstone hung around their neck and to be drowned in the depths of the sea" (NIV).

In this verse, "little ones" doesn't necessarily mean age, but innocence and immaturity as well. For years, I felt like I had been a willing participant instead of a victim. But it wasn't my fault. I never initiated the crime. However, Satan made me think I was a partner in it.

God wanted me released from the chains; therefore, he prompted me to expose this nasty part of my past. I begrudgingly obeyed. The Lord desired to liberate me from this offense and make me whole again. He wanted that foul violation ejected from my heart, so he could place his healing touch on the wound, and he did.

At the time of my emotional healing, I was the mother of three girls under the age of seven. I did not want the effects of my devastating wound influencing them nor did I not want the pattern to continue.

Unhealed emotional wounds leave a hole in a person's heart. We may try to fill that hole with food. I filled it with alcohol. Alcohol became my stronghold because I turned to it instead of God.

Do you turn to food or some other vice to help you deal with stressors of life? If yes, what do you turn to?

_____

_____

Those bad habits are our attempt to put a Band-Aid on our deep hurt. But God is our ultimate healer, not our vice. I am glad I obeyed and exposed my past to my trusted Bible study friends. Exposing my abuse was part of the healing process, and it opened the door to freedom. I was no longer the partner in crime that Satan made me believe I was.

Do you have a deep wound that needs the Lord's healing touch? Are you afraid to expose your secret, like I was? What first step can you take to receive God's healing touch?

_____

_____

Subsequently, I gave my testimony to many groups and at women's retreats. Roman 8:28 was fulfilled: "And we know that God causes everything to work together for the good of those who love God and are called according to his purpose for them." I suffered, but God made right what happened to me, and he can do that for you too. Take the bold step to drag your skeleton out the closet and expose it to Lord's light; this is the key to unlocking the chains of bondage. You will be glad you did.

Are you willing to drag your skeleton out of the closet and share it with the group?

_____

Whether it is abuse or addiction, let's pray the secret offenses be exposed and dealt with appropriately. Emotional wounds such as these can affect our eating behaviors and overall health. We want to improve our bodies from the inside out, so ask God for his healing.

_____

_____

_____

_____

DAY 4: SWORD OF THE SPIRIT

We are more than physical beings; we are spiritual as well. The struggle to get off carbs may not be only a physical battle but a spiritual one too. One of the ways we can fight food addiction is through scripture. Appendix 1 in *7 Steps to Get Off Sugar and Carbohydrates* includes Bible verses to recite to tap into God's power and strength. (You can obtain a printable version of the appendices at http://SusanUNeal.com/appendix.)

If you are addicted to sugar and carbohydrates, you will need his supreme power. Paul tells us in Philippians 4:13, "For I can do everything through Christ, who gives me strength."

An essential component to the arsenal God gave us in Ephesian 6 is the sword of the Spirit:

> Last of all I want to remind you that your strength must come from the Lord's mighty power within you. Put on all of God's armor so that you will be able to stand safe against all strategies and tricks of Satan. For we are not fighting against people made of flesh and blood, but against persons without bodies—the evil rulers of the unseen world, those mighty satanic beings and great evil princes of darkness who

rule this world; and against huge numbers of wicked spirits in the spirit world. So use every piece of God's armor to resist the enemy whenever he attacks, and when it is all over, you will still be standing up. . . .. And you will need the helmet of salvation and the sword of the Spirit—which is the Word of God.

Ephesians 6:10–13, 17, TLB

To use the sword of the Spirit as your weapon, choose a Bible verse that is the opposite of your problem and memorize it. Write the verse on an index card in the following manner: write the verse name and number at the top and bottom of the card. Then break the verse up into short segments that are easy to memorize. For example:

Ephesians 5:18
Don't drink too much wine,
for many evils lie along that path;
be filled instead with the Holy Spirit
and controlled by him.
Ephesians 5:18 (TLB)

This simple and effective method makes it easy to learn one line of the verse at a time. Continue to do this until the entire verse is memorized.

To find a verse, I look in the master index and dictionary/concordance at the back of a Bible. You could look up words like feasting, temptation, or gluttony. Check out the corresponding verses to the different words until you find the one that the Holy Spirit leads you to use. Pray and ask God to help you find the perfect scripture to memorize.

. . .

Memory Verse

Write down the scripture you chose to memorize:

_____

_____

_____

Now write that verse on an index card or in the notes app on your smartphone. Take the scripture card with you on a walk, tape it to the bathroom mirror, or keep it in your purse to review. Be creative! Storing Bible verses in your heart is like storing up treasure, as indicated in Proverbs 2:6, "For the Lord grants wisdom! His every word is a treasure of knowledge and understanding" (TLB).

By storing scriptures in your mind and heart, you can unsheathe the sword of the Spirit at anytime. Speak verses with authority to slash temptations. The spoken Word of God is a double-edged sword that defeats the enemy. Hiding his Word in your heart is vital to your spiritual success on this journey to change. God's Word allows us to know the Holy Spirit better and gain discernment and empowerment. This is crucial to making wise versus foolish choices in every area of life—including food.

DAY 5: TEMPLE OF THE HOLY SPIRIT

"Don't you realize that your body is the temple of the Holy Spirit, who lives in you and was given to you by God? You do not belong to yourself, for God bought you with a high price. So you must honor God with your body" (1 Corinthians 6:19–20). Though this verse in context references sexual immorality, it establishes a foundation for realizing value and ownership.

When you make healthy eating choices, you take care of the temple God gave you. In other words, good self-care honors the Lord. You only have one body, and it needs to last a lifetime. If you are healthy you can fulfill the unique purpose he has planned for you. Also you will be a godly influence in the lives of those you love for a more extended period of time to help them grow into who God created them to be.

In our society it is easy to fall into the *food addiction trap*, and when we do, we are not taking care of our body. Every day we face food temptations. As soon as we take that first bite of a pastry, dopamine releases in the brain, our focus narrows, and we consume more than we planned to eat. Now that you recognize this is a *biochemical addiction*, you can understand yourself better. Food addiction rewires the neural pathways in a person's brain and leads to gluttony.

To prevent gluttonous episodes, track when you overeat in the Binge Eating Tracker in the *Healthy Living Journal*. This chart will help you identify the temptation that triggered the episode. Other physiological symptoms are recorded in this chart so you become aware of the side effects of inappropriate eating. However, there are spiritual implications to overeating as well.

The Bible tells us that gluttony, which is overeating, is a sin, as implied in Proverbs 23:1–3, "When you sit to dine with a ruler, note well what is before you, and put a knife to your throat if you are given to gluttony. Do not crave his delicacies, for that food is deceptive" (NIV).

Deceptive foods tempt us wherever we turn, and we do not have the willpower to stop eating, so we binge. Paul struggled with sin: "The trouble is with me, for I am all too human, a slave to sin. I don't really understand myself, for I want to do what is right, but I don't do it. Instead, I do what I hate" (Romans 7:14–15). Therefore, we cannot fight this battle alone. We need God and his Word.

Do you feel as though you are a slave to something? What?

If you believe you sinned through gluttony, ask God to forgive you and help you overcome the desires of your flesh by writing a prayer below. He will help you, so face the truth without shame and resolve to turn away from any sin.

. . .

With the help of Christ, you can overcome, as Paul expresses in Romans 7:24–25, "Oh, what a miserable person I am! Who will free me from this life that is dominated by sin and death? Thank God! The answer is in Jesus Christ our Lord." Jesus is the key to unlocking the chains of bondage.

Surrender

When we are weak we can become strong through Christ. Let God's power work through you by surrendering your life and issues to Jesus. When you do, you gain access to his power; then you can withstand any temptation. Paul explains this:

> Three different times I begged the Lord to take it away. Each time he said, "My grace is all you need. My power works best in weakness." So now I am glad to boast about my weaknesses so that the power of Christ can work through me. That's why I take pleasure in my weaknesses, and in ... troubles that I suffer for Christ. For when I am weak, then I am strong.
>
> 2 Corinthians 12:8–10

Express to the Lord the struggle you experience with food, then surrender this issue to Jesus.

. . .

Commitment

This week you learned about food addiction, gluttony, and how to fight temptations with the sword of the Spirit. Have you asked someone to be your prayer/accountability partner yet? That is another essential component to your spiritual arsenal. You need these weapons to successfully make the necessary lifestyle changes.

To alter unhealthy eating habits, discredit false beliefs about food by educating yourself. Did you read step 1 in *7 Steps to Get Off Sugar and Carbohydrates*? You won't change unless you understand why it is imperative to transform the way you eat. No more eating food out of a bag or box.

Did the food you want to eat exist in the garden of Eden? If yes, it is beneficial. However, if a food manufacturer transforms a food such as a potato into potato flakes to create "instant mashed potatoes," the food is altered and harmful to the human body. Therefore, evaluate everything you eat and make sure God created it, not the food industry.

Making the decision to commit to a lifestyle change is crucial, particularly if you struggle with food addiction. Remember, no matter if and when you make a mistake, you can get back on track.

. . .

Deciding is the first step to any change. Begin by asking God to make you willing to change. Once you are willing, write down the changes you will make, and commit to them before the Lord. Include the measurable goals you would like to achieve. Ask God to help you and place your success in his loving hands.

Now state in a firm voice (speak out loud) the commitment you just made to God.

Session 1 Action Steps

1. Read the introduction and first chapter (Step 1: Decide to Improve Your Health) in *7 Steps to Get Off Sugar and Carbohydrates.*
2. Acquire a prayer/accountability partner.
3. Request to join the closed Facebook group: 7 Steps to Get Off Sugar and Carbohydrates.
4. Write a commitment between you and God.

5. Don't eat anything with greater than 10 grams of sugar at one sitting.
6. Stop eating refined carbohydrates such as snacks you find in boxes and bags.
7. Take a food addiction test.
8. Drag your skeleton out of the closet and share it with your small group.
9. Write your Bible verse on an index card or under the notes app in your cell phone.
10. Express to God the struggle you experience with food and surrender this issue to Jesus.

PART II

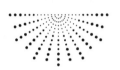

SESSION 2: HARMFUL VERSUS BENEFICIAL FOODS

Last week we learned about food addiction and generational bondage. Today we will explore these topics further by discussing the fill-in-the-blank questions from days 1–5 and the action steps listed at the end of day 5 in session 1. (*Leader: discuss session 1 questions before proceeding.*)

After discussing the questions in session 1, read the second chapter of *7 Steps to Get Off Sugar and Carbohydrates*, Step 2: Acquire a Support System and Knowledge, beginning with the section Harmful Versus Beneficial Foods. Each member can read one paragraph or one section out loud to the group. Whatever portion of the chapter you are not able to finish should be assigned as homework. Ask the following questions after reading each section.

Harmful Versus Beneficial Foods

What was most surprising to you?

. . .

Roundup Ready Crops

Did you know that most of the US wheat, corn, oats, soy, and sugar beet crops were from Roundup Ready seeds? How does this information impact you?

Unhealthy Food Combinations

Can you recall having an upset stomach that might have been caused by a poor food combination? What were the effects on you or your household?

Record digestive issues and the food that may have caused the problem in the Issue Tracker Log in your *Healthy Living Journal*, so you can determine foods that may be inflammatory to your body. Obtain a journal of your own or purchase the *Healthy Living Journal* designed to correspond with this study.

Food Triggers

Are you aware of anything that may initiate an unhealthy eating behavior in yourself? If so, what might that be and what causes this behavior?

. . .

Acquire a Support System

Did you asked someone to be your accountability/prayer partner yet? If yes, who? If not, who are you going to ask and when do you plan to ask them?

Journal

Why is it important to journal your physical and emotional responses to food?

On a daily basis, record the information provided in appendix 3 of *7 Steps to Get Off Sugar and Carbohydrates*. The *Healthy Living Journal* contains all the information.

Scripture

Have you selected the Bible verse you plan to use to fight temptation? Write the verse in the space provided below and on an index card or in the notes app on your smartphone. (*Leader: you could hand out index cards to participants.*)

. . .

(Leader: if time permits, select either the Prayer, Recipe, and/or Scripture Prayer activity below. Each activity should be performed in a smaller group of two to three.)

Prayer

Explain when you struggle with poor eating habits. After sharing, pray for each other and these struggles.

Recipes

While still in your small prayer group, check out appendix 4 in *7 Steps to Get Off Sugar and Carbohydrates* and select a recipe you would like to cook this week. If you have time, plan your menu and grocery list for the week, and encourage each other in this small group as you plan. For healthy menus, recipes, and grocery lists check out Susan-UNeal.com/healthy-living-blog.

Scripture Prayer

Praying is a vital component of our spiritual arsenal. Prayer and the sword of the Spirit are our two offensive weapons. Use them often and combine them. Ask each person in the small group to recite (out loud) the Scripture verse they chose and create a prayer from it (space is provided below). If someone does not feel comfortable speaking, she may write out her prayer. For example, the Bible verse I selected is, "Don't drink too much wine, for many evils lie along that path; be filled instead with the Holy Spirit and controlled by him" Ephesians 5:18 (TLB).

My prayer is: *Dear heavenly father, I want to be controlled by the Holy Spirit, not by my desire to consume an alcoholic beverage or anything else that is unhealthy for me. Please help me be mindful that your Spirit resides in my body—it is the temple of the Holy Spirit—so I should be a good steward of my body. Please help me be controlled by your Spirit, not by my fleshly desires. Through Jesus's name, I pray. Amen.*

Write your scripture prayer below:

Conclusion

Beware of corn, wheat, oat, soy, and beet products because most crops in the United States are Roundup Ready crops so they may have the carcinogenic residue of glyphosate. Therefore, eat only organic products from these five different foods. Also avoid eating wheat or consuming more than 10 grams of sugar in one serving.

As a group, decide whether you want to read the third chapter of *7 Steps to Get Off Sugar and Carbohydrates*, Step 3: Clean Out the Pantry and Refrigerator, on your own or during session 3.

DAY 1: CANDIDA

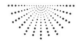

Read the section titled Understanding Candida in chapter 2 of *7 Steps to Get Off Sugar and Carbohydrates*. A list of symptoms that are indicative of a candida infection is provided. You completed the same symptom checklist in session 1. Count how many signs you experience and write that number here _____.

The more symptoms you experience, the more likely you have an overgrowth of Candida. God created our gastrointestinal systems with a perfect balance of yeast and beneficial microorganisms. However, antibiotics kill the beneficial ones, and most people do not know to take probiotics after they finish a course of antibiotics. Consequently, the yeast starts to grow and take over.

People who have taken antibiotics numerous times in their lives should take a probiotic supplement. There are many different strains of beneficial microbes, but we don't know which ones we need unless we have an expensive stool analysis performed. In lieu of this test, purchase a probiotic with at least ten strains of microorganisms. When you run out, buy a different brand, so you don't repeat the same variety. That way you reculture your gut with varying types of probiotics generally found in a healthy GI tract.

To determine if you have an overgrowth of Candida, perform the spit test described in step 2 of *7 Steps to Get Off Sugar and Carbohydrates*. Tomorrow, when you wake up, complete the spit test. It might be convenient to place a glass of water in your bathroom the night before since you should not drink or brush your teeth before you spit in the cup.

Did your saliva have strings hanging down? Answer here _____. If yes, purchase an anti-Candida cleanse to take when you get to session 5, where more information is provided.

DAY 2: HUMILITY

In day 1 we discussed how to obtain a balance in the GI tract. Today we will focus internally—not on the physical body but the soul. Attaining a balance between humility and pride may be just as challenging as balancing the gut.

A healthy ego embraces a positive attitude toward our talents and God-given gifts. It is natural to feel proud sentiments about an accomplishment or meeting a goal. Similarly, we hope to achieve many goals through this study. The Lord wants us to have a positive self-image and feel confident about ourselves. Therefore, when kept in balance, pride can be healthy; however, when we think we are better than others, we are out of balance. That is similar to Candida in our gut. When in balance, the Candida's presence in our bodies is the way God made us, but when it flourishes out of control, it takes over —like pride.

Humility is part of Lord's upside-down world. One might think pride would bring honor, and humility humiliation, but the opposite is true. "Pride ends in humiliation, while humility brings honor" (Proverbs 29:23).

The Lord appreciates humility as it is expressed through being courteous and respectful of others, and not thinking of yourself as better than anyone else. Jesus told his twelve disciples in Mark 9:35, "Whoever wants to be first must take last place and be the servant of everyone else." Humility sees the dignity and worth of every human being. Being humble does not mean we should deny our self-worth; as children of God, we are entitled to all the blessings he planned for us.

On the other hand, a prideful person won't admit his faults or sins. He puts his confidence in his power and abilities, not God's. Pride is like having a stone cover a person's heart, so the ugliness within won't be exposed. Prideful people choose to keep their secrets in the dark and pretend they are perfect. They won't reveal their heart to the Lord; therefore, they can't be forgiven nor healed of their wounds.

Do you have a secret you need to reveal to God? Write down your confession to him.

_____

_____

If you have a wound that needs healing, ask the Lord to heal it.

_____

_____

A form of pride occurs when we become self-absorbed. We obsess about our looks, illness, weight—you name it. If we take our focus off ourselves and pay attention to God, noneternal things will not preoccupy us or entice us to sin.

Another area of pride arises when we think we can't forgive ourselves because we believe our sin is too big or evil. God is greater than our sin, and in his eyes, all sin is sin. He can forgive anyone who is genuinely sorry for what they did, no matter what it was. All one needs to do is sincerely ask for forgiveness. It's that simple.

Pride is the desire to exalt oneself above others, whereas a low self-esteem is lacking confidence. An individual may believe she is inadequate, unlovable, and incompetent. However, God loves each of us immensely, and everyone deserves to be treated with respect. Some people are prone to pride, while others suffer from low self-esteem. Leaning in one direction or the other does not characterize a healthy ego.

Do you lean toward being prideful or having a low self-esteem? Either way, how does this affect your life?

To achieve a better balance, what steps can you take?

.   .   .

What does a healthy ego look like? A person with a healthy ego gives glory to God instead of himself. When we feel weak or not good enough, we should ask the Lord to help us, and invite his power and strength to enable us to withstand the trials and temptations we face. When we are victorious, we should give him the glory.

What victory have you achieved when God helped you?

God gives strength to the humble but sets himself against the proud and haughty. So give yourselves humbly to God. Resist the devil and he will flee from you. And when you draw close to God, God will draw close to you.

James 4:6–8 (TLB)

Write a scripture prayer by using the verse above.

DAY 3: PRIDE IN THE LAST DAYS

Pride leads people to be self-centered and conclude they deserve everything they want. It creates a greedy appetite. Fortunately, God releases us from our selfish desires when we humble ourselves before him. Becoming humble and relying on the Lord is the cure for pride, just like an anti-Candida cleanse is the cure for an overgrowth of this type of yeast.

James 4:6–7 tells us that when we submit to God, he gives us his strength to resist the devil, and Satan will go away. Humility helps us recognize our weaknesses and believe God can strengthen and improve them.

Write down a weakness you would like the Lord to strengthen, and pray, asking him to help you improve it.

. . .

When we are humble, we recognize how small we are in comparison to the Lord's greatness. Every day we have to decide whether to follow God's commands and his Holy Spirit's guidance in our life. If we choose to talk to him throughout the day, like a friend, he will support us during our challenges. Tapping into his power often will help us make better choices.

We live in a self-centered, excessive culture. The sights and scents of succulent unhealthy, foods tempt us everywhere we turn. The enticing world of moral decay calls us. Yet if we want to live for the Lord, we must purposefully resist worldly temptations.

What worldly things tempt you?

Praying and asking for God's assistance reminds us that we can't stay in his will without his help. Many times we look for help from other people, things, or substances. But all the time the Lord yearns for us to ask him for help. When we do, we will obtain the strength we need.

Do you turn to worldly things for help rather than God? If yes, what?

. . .

Paul warns us in 2 Timothy 3:15 of the dangers of the last days:

You should know this, Timothy, that in the last days there will be very difficult times. For people will love only themselves and their money. They will be boastful and proud, scoffing at God, disobedient to their parents, and ungrateful. They will consider nothing sacred. They will be unloving and unforgiving; they will slander others and have no self-control. They will be cruel and hate what is good. They will betray their friends, be reckless, be puffed up with pride, and love pleasure rather than God. They will act religious, but they will reject the power that could make them godly. Stay away from people like that!

Paul may be talking about an overinflated ego or narcissism. Narcissism is the love of oneself with a corresponding lack of feeling or interest for other people. This type of egotism is becoming a more common flaw in our society.

The cause of narcissism is not known for sure, but one scientific theory links it to deep, childhood, emotional wounding from various forms of abuse, which elicits shame or humiliation in the child.[1] The injury stunts the child's emotional development. Therefore, they do not develop a healthy sense of self. Instead, they feel entitled and think the whole world should revolve around their needs and desires. The least bit of criticism is interpreted as rejection. They can't accept their flaws, so they hide them. They crave constant praise and do not consider the wishes of others.

Do you know someone with narcissistic traits? How does this affect their relationship with you or others?

———

. . .

A humble person courageously acknowledges the damage done to him or her in childhood and trusts that God can heal it. We want to heal from the inside out because emotional wounds affect our physical, emotional, and mental well-being.

Place before the Lord your childhood wounds and ask him to heal you.

When we humble ourselves before the Lord, we can be assured that he will heal us and help us become a better person—more humble, less prideful. In this way we tap into God's strength and are empowered to follow him.

DAY 4: KING SAUL'S PRIDE

In day 3 we compared Candida to pride. When the balance between the beneficial microorganisms and this form of yeast is balanced, the gastrointestinal system is healthy. The same is true when we have a positive self-esteem, yet are humble and rely on God. However, the overgrowth of either pride or Candida creates an unhealthy environment. Today we will explore pride within the human ego and see how the deflation and inflation of Saul's pride caused his demise.

Saul's story began when he tried to find his dad's lost donkeys. The donkey quest led him to the prophet Samuel's home. God spoke to Samuel the previous day and told him:

"About this time tomorrow I will send you a man from the land of Benjamin. Anoint him to be the leader of my people, Israel. He will rescue them from the Philistines, for I have looked down on my people in mercy and have heard their cry." When Samuel saw Saul, the LORD said, "That's the man I told you about! He will rule my people."

1 Samuel 9:15–17

During Saul's unexpected visit, Samuel anointed Saul as king. "Then Samuel took a flask of olive oil and poured it over Saul's head. He kissed Saul and said, 'I am doing this because the LORD has appointed you to be the ruler over Israel, his special possession'" (1 Samuel 10:1). Sometime later:

> Samuel brought all the tribes of Israel before the LORD, and the tribe of Benjamin was chosen by lot. Then he brought each family of the tribe of Benjamin before the LORD, and the family of the Matrites was chosen. And finally Saul son of Kish was chosen from among them. But when they looked for him, he had disappeared! So they asked the LORD, "Where is he?" And the LORD replied, "He is hiding among the baggage." So they found him and brought him out, and he stood head and shoulders above anyone else.
>
> 1 Samuel 10:20–23

Why in the world would Saul hide as he is being chosen as the king of Israel? It doesn't make sense; neither does the human ego. The natural inclination of the ego is for it to become inflated and deflated.[2] Naturally, we care about what other people think of us, and our ego is boosted when we are complimented or achieve success. Sadly, most people do not stay content for long because the human ego cannot be satisfied; it always wants more.

The ego craves attention; it wants to be puffed up—complimented and noticed. Unfortunately, what gets puffed up must come down, and when that occurs, as in the case of someone having something better, a person may feel deflated. The inflation and deflation of the ego become an emotional roller coaster.

. . .

Do you know someone whose moods consistently reflect an emotional roller coaster?

Saul's ego must have been inflated after Samuel anointed him during their first meeting. What happened that deflated his ego to the point of hiding when he knew he was about to be officially chosen as king before the people? Did he not believe that he would be selected? Was he afraid of failure or what others would think of him? Interestingly, after he was initially anointed, he didn't tell anyone. Maybe he thought he wouldn't be a suitable king, or he had no idea how to proceed when he was chosen.

The next situation in Saul's life demonstrates a complete over inflation of his ego:

Saul waited seven days for Samuel, as Samuel had instructed him earlier, but Samuel still didn't come. Saul realized that his troops were rapidly slipping away. So he demanded, "Bring me the burnt offering and the peace offerings!" And Saul sacrificed the burnt offering himself.

Just as Saul was finishing with the burnt offering, Samuel arrived. Saul went out to meet and welcome him, but Samuel said, "What is this you have done?"

Saul replied, "I saw my men scattering from me, and you didn't arrive when you said you would, and the Philistines are at Micmash ready for battle. So I said, 'The Philistines are ready to march against us at Gilgal, and I haven't even asked for the LORD's help!' So I felt compelled to offer the burnt offering myself before you came."

"How foolish!" Samuel exclaimed. "You have not kept the command the LORD your God gave you. Had you kept it, the LORD would have established your kingdom over Israel forever. But now your kingdom must end, for the LORD has sought out a man after his own heart. The LORD has already appointed him to be the leader of his people, because you have not kept the LORD's command."

1 Samuel 13:8–14

Samuel had given King Saul specific instructions to wait for him to offer the sacrifices. But fear gripped Saul's heart as he saw his troops slipping away. Time was running out. At that point he should have gotten down on his knees and prayed.

Instead, Saul "demanded" that the offerings be brought to him. God's laws forbid anyone other than a priest to offer sacrifices. So what did Saul do? He did the unthinkable. He substituted himself as a priest.

A few minutes after Saul offered the sacrifice, Samuel showed up. Saul greeted him and acted as if he had done nothing wrong. On day 3 we talked about a narcissistic trait: when a person who has done wrong doesn't think he has done anything wrong. Saul couldn't accept his mistake, so he covered it up with excuses: "You didn't arrive when you said you would." He blamed Samuel.

King Saul's justification and excuses were nothing more than disobedience to Samuel and God's law. It didn't take long for the first king of Israel to disobey and lose the inheritance of his kingdom that could have been passed down to his descendants. Forty years later, David finally became the king.

Can you think of a situation when you blamed others instead of accepting responsibility for your actions? What did you feel like at the time? Did you have remorse or regret? What were the consequences of your excuses and blame?

. . .

I was a blamer. I found any excuse to blame something or someone else instead of myself. I realized that my mother also had this trait, and I learned that behavior from her. I wanted to eliminate this character flaw, and instead, emulate Christ. When we recognize our imperfections we can go to the Lord and ask him to empower us to change.

Write a prayer and ask God to perfect your imperfections.

.   .   .

DAY 5: IDENTITY IN CHRIST

King Saul's pride led him to be disobedient, which caused disastrous consequences. Because of his disobedience, his son, Jonathan, would never take the throne. God wanted a humble, obedient, servant king, not an egotistical one.

How does one cure the insatiable appetite of the human ego? Paul tells us how in 1 Corinthians 4:3–4: "I care very little if I am judged by you or by any human court; indeed, I do not even judge myself. My conscience is clear, but that does not make me innocent. It is the Lord who judges me" (NIV). When we care more about what God thinks of us, and not what other people think, it cures us of the emotional roller coaster of an inflated and deflated ego.

Paul did not care if other people "judged" him. He knew the Lord judges. When we stop caring about our image, but instead care about what the Lord thinks of our character, we eliminate the need to seek external approval. It doesn't matter what the next-door neighbor believes; God knows the intentions of our hearts. He alone is the judge; we are not.

What relief we feel when we don't have to "keep up with the Joneses." Status, fame, and worldly concerns slip away. Instead, we get our approval from one source—God—who loves us enough to send his one and only son to die for us.

Our identity is in Jesus Christ and the sacrifice he made for us. We get off the emotional roller coaster when we do not link our identity to our accomplishments or sins. Christ took our sins upon himself when he died on the cross, so we would be made holy and clean before God. Now we are part of his family, and "Therefore, there is now no condemnation for those who are in Christ Jesus" (Romans 8:1 NIV). What a relief to know that we will not be condemned when we go to heaven, because Jesus was condemned for us, and he received our punishment.

It doesn't matter what you think of yourself, because you become transformed as you trust Jesus to take away your sins—to be the sacrificial lamb that died for you. Once you accept Christ as your Lord and Savior and follow him, he becomes your new identity. "For we are to God the pleasing aroma of Christ" (2 Corinthians 2:15 NIV). God even thinks we smell like his son!

Ask the Lord to exchange the desire you have for the world's approval, for his approval.

_____

_____

_____

When we are not concerned with what others think of us, or even what we think of ourselves, but instead focus on what God thinks, we arrive at humility. Timothy Keller, author of *The Freedom of Self-*

Forgetfulness, wrote, "The essence of gospel-humility is not thinking more of myself or thinking less of myself, it is thinking of myself less."[3] Instead of worrying about how you look or focusing on your weight, you should think less about yourself altogether. Focus on who you are in Christ.

Describe the difference it would make in your life and relationships if you focused on what God thinks of you instead of what you or others may think.

_____

_____

Session 2 Action Steps

1. Read the second chapter of *7 Steps to Get Off Sugar and Carbohydrates*, titled Step 2: Acquire a Support System and Knowledge.
2. Plan your menu and grocery list for the week.
3. Only eat organic corn, wheat, oat, soy, and beet products because of the potential carcinogenic glyphosate residue.
4. Avoid eating wheat.
5. Record your food and activity for this week in the *Healthy Living Journal.*
6. Conduct the Candida spit test. If it is positive, purchase an anti-Candida cleanse.

PART III

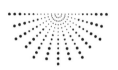

SESSION 3: CLEAN OUT YOUR EMOTIONS

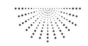

Last week we learned that Candida and unhealthy foods could harm us physically, whereas, pride can harm us spiritually. Today we will review these topics further by discussing the fill-in-the-blank questions from days 1–5 and the action steps listed at the end of day 5 in session 2. (*Leader: discuss session 2 questions before proceeding.*)

Prayer

Praying for one another is an essential component of our spiritual arsenal. Therefore, after discussing last week's questions, pray for each other, as some members may have exposed their skeletons for the first time.

Next read the third chapter of *7 Steps to Get Off Sugar and Carbohydrates*, titled Step 3: Clean Out the Pantry and Refrigerator. Stop reading at the section "Clean Out Your Emotions." Each member can read one paragraph or section out loud to the group. Whatever portion of the chapter you are not able to finish should be assigned as homework. Ask the following questions after reading this chapter. (*Note*: Participants should watch on their own the documentary The

Sugar Film and "What's in Your Pantry," video by Dr. Daniel Amen at: Youtube.com/watch?v=VqoWO0-RSAI.[1])

Food to Eliminate

Place an X by the food you think will be most difficult to eliminate from your diet and as a group discuss why.

_____ wheat

_____ white flour

_____ sugar

_____ corn syrup

_____ white rice

_____ corn

_____ milk products

_____ artificial sweeteners

_____ processed meats

_____ vegetable oils

_____ processed foods

_____ peanuts

_____ canned goods

_____ margarine

From the list above, what food (that you need to avoid) surprised you the most?

_____

I had no idea that processed meats were a carcinogen, did you? What type of processed meats do you primarily eat? How do you plan to avoid them in the future?

. . .

Clean Out the Pantry

What type of foods do you primarily need to remove from the pantry?

Clean Out the Refrigerator

Have you ever thought about the ingredients in condiments? Does it surprise you that many contain unhealthy ingredients?

Clean Out Your Freezer

What products do you plan to try in place of ice cream? Have you ever tasted a nondairy ice cream?

Do you think it will be more difficult to clean out your pantry, refrigerator, or freezer? Why?

. . .

Clean Out Your Emotions

Do you engage in emotional or stress eating? What usually initiates the eating behavior?

_____

Do you think it will be more difficult to clean out your cupboards or emotions? Why?

_____

Did you find it surprising that bisphenol (BPA) lined the inside of canned goods, and consumers who eat food out of cans have this chemical passed through our bodies and into their urine? Do you plan to avoid canned foods in the future?

_____

Plan Ahead to Avoid Emotional and Stress Eating

How can you plan ahead to avoid emotional or stress eating?

_____

_____

_____

. . .

Conclusion

We will be cleaning out our cupboards this week, so end your session in prayer by asking God to help members make wise decisions and be motivated to change. As a group, decide whether you want to read the fourth chapter of *7 Steps to Get Off Sugar and Carbohydrates*, Step 4: Purchase Healthy Foods and Anti-Candida Cleanse, on your own or during session 4.

DAY 1: CLEAN OUT THE PANTRY, REFRIGERATOR, AND FREEZER

This week we will be cleaning out the pantry, refrigerator, and freezer. Start by watching the fifteen-minute video by Dr. Daniel Amen who coauthored *The Daniel Plan*. Watch "What's in Your Pantry" at: Youtube.com/watch?v=VqoWO0-RSAI.[2]

Schedule a date to clean out your pantry, refrigerator, and freezer.

Date to clean out:

Pantry _____

Refrigerator _____

Freezer _____

Clean Out the Pantry
Remove the following unhealthy items from your pantry:

- Wheat—anything that contains wheat
- Sugar-sweetened drinks—like soda, fruit juice, Gatorade
- Sugar—white sugar, high-fructose corn syrup—remove any item with greater than ten grams of sugar per serving. (Unfortunately, sugar does not have a recommended daily allowance.)
- Rice—white rice (brown and wild rice are fine)
- Corn—all nonorganic corn products such as tortilla chips and popcorn (Organic corn products are fine to consume.)
- Artificial sweeteners—saccharin, aspartame or Equal/NutraSweet, sucralose or Splenda (It is okay to keep honey, maple syrup, agave, stevia, xylitol, coconut sugar, and monk fruit sugar.)
- Oils—eliminate all oils except olive oil (use when cooking at low temperatures) and coconut oil (use when cooking at high temperatures)
- Any processed food in a box or bag such as chips, crackers, cookies, and cereal (unless it is organic and you choose to make this an exception)
- Foods that contain partially hydrogenated vegetable oil, high-fructose corn syrup, or monosodium glutamate (MSG)

Clean Out the Refrigerator

Let's move on to cleaning out the refrigerator. Remove the following unhealthy items from your refrigerator:

- Wheat products
- Processed meats such as ham, bacon, sausage, hot dogs, and lunch meat
- Soft drinks and fruit juices—they are loaded with sugar

- Check the ingredients of condiments. If one contains high-fructose corn syrup, throw it out. Health-food stores carry better condiment substitutes, such as organic mayonnaise.
- Margarine—organic butter is a healthier choice
- All milk products except plain Greek yogurt, which contains probiotics

Clean Out Your Freezer

Next let's open up that freezer and see what is inside. Throw out the following unhealthy products:

- Wheat products
- Dairy products (Replace your dairy products, such as ice cream, with coconut, almond, or cashew milk items.)
- Packaged frozen meals (while convenient, even the "healthy" brands of frozen foods are processed)

What an incredible accomplishment to clean out these areas of your kitchen. Now unhealthy foods will no longer tempt you. Congratulations!

DAY 2: CLEAN OUT YOUR EMOTIONS

Now that we cleaned out the pantry, refrigerator, and freezer, it is time to clean out our emotions. What do emotions have to do with eating? Possible nothing, or it could be the root cause of a dysfunctional eating behavior. Please read the section titled "Clean Out Your Emotions" in the third chapter (Step 3: Clean Out the Pantry and Refrigerator) of *7 Steps to Get Off Sugar and Carbohydrates*.

Do you have a specific comfort food you enjoy? For me, it is popcorn. However, I try to improve the nutritional value of this snack by using heirloom, organic kernels and sprinkling it with sea salt and seaweed (dulse and kelp seaweed sprinkles). As seen in Genesis 3:4–7, Eve found the forbidden fruit "pleasing to the eye." Eve saw that the fruit looked delicious and she desired it. Do you ever desire an appealing dessert? I know I do. I enjoy tiramisu, and fight the temptation to eat it.

What foods do you find pleasing to the eye? What appeals to you about these foods?

. . .

Do you ever turn to food instead of God to help you cope? Why do you think you do this?

What type of emotions do you experience when you turn to food? Does the food satiate your emotions?

It is imperative to document why you choose to eat in your *Healthy Living Journal*. Do you want to eat because you are hungry or is there an emotional component to your desire? Journaling will help you connect the dots between your eating habits and emotions. In your journal, record your thoughts as they relate to your consumption of food. Are you eating because of a negative emotion? Figure out what triggers you to eat (when you are not hungry). This may help you identify dysfunctional eating behaviors. Don't treat these symptoms with a trendy new diet. Instead, determine the root cause, deal with it, and seek healing.

What do you think is the root cause of your unhealthy eating habits?

_____

_____

_____

After you pinpoint your issue with food, bring it to God and be honest with him about what you experience. Each time you recognize that you engage in emotional eating, clean out your emotions with the Lord so you can disengage the connection between eating and feelings.

Begin the process of cleaning out your emotions with God by telling him what you think is the origin of your unhealthy eating habit and ask him to help you heal from any emotional scars.

_____

_____

_____

. . .

_____

Have you tried to overcome inappropriate eating before? If you failed, you were probably dealing with the issue through your own resolve. Instead, call on the power of the Holy Spirit to change you from the inside out. With God's help, you can overcome and succeed.

Write your prayer below asking the Lord to help you overcome any eating challenges you may face.

_____

_____

_____

_____

DAY 3: ACCESS GOD'S POWER

Have you ever relied on self-control to overcome temptations of the flesh but failed? Instead, we need to use God's power to conquer food issues. How do we access his power? Let's look for the answer in the Bible. Speak these verses out loud:

In your hands are strength and power to exalt and give strength to all.

1 Chronicles 29:12 (NIV)

You are their glorious strength. It pleases you to make us strong.

Psalm 89:17

The eyes of the LORD search the whole earth in order to strengthen those whose hearts are fully committed to him.

2 Chronicles 16:9

From these verses, we see that "the Lord" can "give strength to all" and it pleases him "to make us strong." He even searches the whole earth to "strengthen those whose hearts are fully committed to him."

What does it mean to you to fully commit your heart to God?

_____

_____

Fully committing means we follow God's rules and let him lead our lives. We accomplish this through obeying his Word and paying attention to the prompting of the Holy Spirit inside of us. To become closer to the Lord we should pray throughout the day, not just at bedtime or before meals. For example, before you get out of bed each morning, say hello to the Lord and ask him to be with you throughout your day. As the day progresses, remain in contact with him spiritually through talking to him and asking for his help and guidance as you need it. Nothing is too small or big for you to converse with him about. He wants to be a part of your life, but you need to let him in.

It is important to spend time with God, maybe through reading a devotion or a Bible verse, as well as spending meditative time in his presence. Ask him to lead you and he will. Through salvation, we received the Holy Spirit. Receiving God's Spirit is like a seed, which needs soil, sunlight, water, and fertilizer to grow. As the seed grows, so does our ability to access his power through the Spirit. The following four habits can help you fully commit your life to the Lord:

. . .

1. Submit (soil) control of your life to Jesus by asking him to lead your life. Ask him for guidance in the small and large decisions. Pray that the choices you make will be in God's will. Write your prayer below.

_____

_____

_____

2. Study and memorize scripture verses (sunlight). What Bible verse do you want to memorize? Write it here:

_____

_____

3. Spend time (water) with the Lord. A section in the *Healthy Living Journal*, the Well-Being Chart helps you track whether you are spending time with God on a daily basis, so you can see if allotting time for God decreases your binging and consumption of unhealthy food.

4. Fellowship (fertilizer) with other Christians through taking a Bible study, attending Sunday school or a small group, or going to Wednesday evening prayer services. How are you socializing with

other Christians? If you are not fellowshipping, how do you plan to incorporate this into your life?

Is your heart fully committed to God? If yes, how is this demonstrated in your life? If no, what steps will you take to fully commit yourself to him?

Psalm 89:17 states that it pleases God to make us strong. So ask him to give you his supernatural strength to make healthy eating choices and not fall prey to temptations. Compose your prayer:

When you are tempted to eat unhealthy foods, remember to recite your Bible verse that opposes your food issue. Have you memorized this verse yet? It is your sword; carry it with you.

DAY 4: STRESS EATING

Stress also causes us to turn to food instead of God. Determine the stressors (things that cause you stress) in your life, and list them below. Evaluate each one and brainstorm on how to minimize them. Pray to the Lord and ask him to enlighten and help you.

Stressor/How to Decrease

_____

_____

_____

_____

. . .

After you brainstorm and pray, call your accountability partner and ask her to pray with you to appropriately deal with the things that cause you stress. Also journal when you engage in stress eating, so you can continue to connect the dots between stress and emotional eating.

Please read the sections titled Plan Ahead to Avoid Emotional and Stress Eating and Taking Step 3: Clean Out in the third chapter (Step 3: Clean Out the Pantry and Refrigerator) of *7 Steps to Get Off Sugar and Carbohydrates.*

How do you cope with stress? Some stress-relieving activities include praying with your prayer partner, enjoying a massage, journaling, and exercising.

Do you engage in stress-relieving activities? If yes, please list them.

_____

_____

If not, what actions do you plan to incorporate into your life to relieve your stress?

_____

_____

Mindfulness exercises such as Christian yoga and meditation train a person to pay attention to cravings without reacting to them. Learn to be proactive rather than reactive to stress. The idea is to ride out the wave of intense desire. As a person becomes more mindful, she notices why she wants to indulge. Meditation quiets the part of the brain that can lead to a loop of obsession.[3] I created several Christian yoga products including DVDs, books, and card decks, available at ChristianYoga.com, that could help you become more mindful.

DAY 5: FORGIVENESS

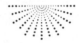

Another component of emotional healing is forgiving those who hurt us or our loved ones. I needed to forgive my perpetrator. Without forgiving him, my wound would not completely heal. The biblical character Joseph also needed to forgive his brothers who sold him into slavery.

The story of Joseph began as Rachel (Jacob's favorite wife) finally gave birth to Joseph, after many years of being barren. Jacob spoiled Joseph, and it was apparent to everyone that Joseph was his father's favorite son—though he already had ten sons when Joseph was born.

When Joseph was a teenager, he dreamed that all his brothers, mother, and father would bow to him. His brothers were offended by the dream and jealous of a beautiful robe Jacob gave Joseph. Therefore, Joseph's brothers plotted to kill him:

> When Joseph's brothers saw him coming, they recognized him in the distance. As he approached, they made plans to kill him. "Here comes the dreamer!" they said. "Come on, let's kill him and throw him into one of these cisterns. We can tell our father, 'A wild animal has eaten him.' Then we'll see what becomes of his dreams!"

But when Reuben heard of their scheme, he came to Joseph's rescue. "Let's not kill him," he said. "Why should we shed any blood? Let's just throw him into this empty cistern here in the wilderness. Then he'll die without our laying a hand on him." Reuben was secretly planning to rescue Joseph and return him to his father.

So when Joseph arrived, his brothers ripped off the beautiful robe he was wearing. Then they grabbed him and threw him into the cistern. Now the cistern was empty; there was no water in it. Then, just as they were sitting down to eat, they looked up and saw a caravan of camels in the distance coming toward them. It was a group of Ishmaelite traders taking a load of gum, balm, and aromatic resin from Gilead down to Egypt.

Judah said to his brothers, "What will we gain by killing our brother? We'd have to cover up the crime. Instead of hurting him, let's sell him to those Ishmaelite traders. After all, he is our brother—our own flesh and blood!" And his brothers agreed.

Genesis 37:18–27

His brothers sold Joseph for twenty pieces of silver. Joseph endured significant hardship in Egypt, including being a slave in Potiphar's home and a prisoner because Potiphar's wife falsely accused Joseph of rape.

I wonder what emotions Joseph felt toward his brothers during those years of hardship. However, God gave Joseph the ability to interpret dreams, and he interpreted Pharaoh's dream about a seven-year famine:

"But afterward there will be seven years of famine so great that all the prosperity will be forgotten in Egypt. Famine will destroy the land. This famine will be so severe that even the memory of the good years will be erased. As for having two similar dreams, it means that these events have been decreed by God, and he will soon make them happen.

Therefore, Pharaoh should find an intelligent and wise man and put him in charge of the entire land of Egypt. Then Pharaoh should appoint supervisors over the land and let them collect one-fifth of all the crops during the seven good years. Have them gather all the food produced in the good years that are just ahead and bring it to Pharaoh's storehouses. Store it away, and guard it so there will be food in the cities. That way there will be enough to eat when the seven years of famine come to the land of Egypt. Otherwise this famine will destroy the land."

Joseph's suggestions were well received by Pharaoh and his officials. So Pharaoh asked his officials, "Can we find anyone else like this man so obviously filled with the spirit of God?" Then Pharaoh said to Joseph, "Since God has revealed the meaning of the dreams to you, clearly no one else is as intelligent or wise as you are. You will be in charge of my court, and all my people will take orders from you. Only I, sitting on my throne, will have a rank higher than yours."

Pharaoh said to Joseph, "I hereby put you in charge of the entire land of Egypt." Then Pharaoh removed his signet ring from his hand and placed it on Joseph's finger. He dressed him in fine linen clothing and hung a gold chain around his neck.

Genesis 41:30–42

In one swift move, Joseph went from being a prisoner to second-in-command of Egypt. By this time Joseph had been estranged from his family for over a decade.

During the famine, Joseph's brothers came to Egypt for food. Ultimately, his father, Jacob, and his brothers came to live in Egypt, and their family was reunited. Read Genesis 42–45 for the full story.

Several years later, when Jacob died, his brothers believed Joseph would seek revenge against them, but he had forgiven them. The betrayal was not forgotten, but he did not want restitution:

> So they sent this message to Joseph: "Before your father died, he instructed us to say to you: 'Please forgive your brothers for the great wrong they did to you—for their sin in treating you so cruelly.' So we, the servants of the God of your father, beg you to forgive our sin." When Joseph received the message, he broke down and wept. Then his brothers came and threw themselves down before Joseph. "Look, we are your slaves!" they said.
>
> But Joseph replied, "Don't be afraid of me. Am I God, that I can punish you? You intended to harm me, but God intended it all for good. He brought me to this position so I could save the lives of many people. No, don't be afraid. I will continue to take care of you and your children." So he reassured them by speaking kindly to them.

Genesis 50:16–21

I find it intriguing that Joseph "broke down and wept" when he received his brothers' message. Did he weep because he remembered when his brothers threw him in the cistern and sold him into slavery? Or could it be because it hurt his heart when he realized they thought he wanted revenge when he held no bitterness in his heart toward them?

Would you like to take revenge against someone who harmed you or your loved one? If yes, how would you carry out your revenge?

_____

. . .

Paul tells us in Romans 12:19, "Dear friends, never take revenge. Leave that to the righteous anger of God. For the Scriptures say, 'I will take revenge; I will pay them back,' says the LORD." God's revenge is worse than what our revenge would be. The consequences that happened in my perpetrator's life are unbelievable, far worse than what I envisioned. The eternal punishment our offenders may receive is endless.

Instead of revenge God calls us to forgive. Jesus talks about forgiveness in Matthew 6:14–15: "For if you forgive other people when they sin against you, your heavenly Father will also forgive you. But if you do not forgive others their sins, your Father will not forgive your sins" (NIV). If we don't forgive others, then God won't forgive us. That is a huge price to pay to hold on to an offense.

Yet it is a process to forgive someone. For me, when I realized I was not a willing participant but a victim, my heart seethed with fury. I experienced anger for the wrong that was done to me. But over the course of a year, I told my husband and another Bible study group, and I even spoke at a women's retreat. Through taking my skeleton out of the closet and sharing with others, I processed the hurt.

A year after I first told the Women of the Word Bible study group about my abuse as a youth, I spoke to my perpetrator. He was about to have major surgery. I wished him well and told him I would pray for him. When I hung up the phone, I did not harbor hard feelings in my heart. The hurt, anger, and desire for revenge were gone—those negative emotions no longer plagued me. I was free. I hope you can become free of any wrongdoings done against you too.

Do you want to be freed from hard feelings in your heart? Describe the negative emotions you experience.

. . .

Another remarkable point Joseph told his brothers was, "You intended to harm me, but God intended it all for good." Similarly, through sharing my testimony, I hope to help others process their hurts and forgive those who harmed them. Maybe after you heal, you can help others, and Romans 8:28 will ring true for you: "And we know that God causes everything to work together for the good of those who love God and are called according to his purpose for them."

Do you need to forgive someone? If yes, then complete one of the activities below to help you forgive:

1. Write a letter to the person you need to forgive. Pour out your feelings on the page. This person may no longer be alive or you may not want to give the letter to this person. To signify the release of your forgiveness, bury or burn the letter.
2. Have a pretend conversation with your offender. This is what I did twenty-five years after the abuse. Even though the person who harmed me was still alive, I did not want to confront this non-Christian man. Instead, I pretended he was sitting in front of me, and I let him have it. I told him what he did to me was sickening, and he was a vile person. I yelled at him and cried. I poured my emotions upon this imaginary figure. It is hard to express the depth of the healing I received from this experience.
3. Create a prayer below asking God to help you forgive.

· · ·

Please consider sharing your forgiveness story with your small group. I can't express how instrumental sharing my story with others helped me to heal.

Dear heavenly Father, please help (insert your name) *forgive whoever harmed her. Please make something good come out of something bad. In Jesus's name, I pray. Amen.*

Session 3 Action Steps

1. Read the third chapter of *7 Steps to Get Off Sugar and Carbohydrates*, Step 3: Clean Out the Pantry and Refrigerator.
2. Clean out your pantry, refrigerator, and freezer.
3. Clean out your emotions with God by telling him what you think is the origin of your unhealthy eating habits and ask him to help you heal from any emotional scars.
4. Fully commit your heart to the Lord.
5. Determine the stressors (things that cause you stress) in your life, and figure out how to minimize them.
6. If you need to forgive someone, complete one of the activities suggested in day 5.
7. Share your forgiveness story with your small group.

PART IV

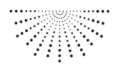

SESSION 4: PURCHASE HEALTHY FOOD

Congratulations on making it halfway through the study. You completed a great deal of work, from determining if you have an overgrowth of Candida to cleaning out your pantry and fridge. In this session you will find out which foods are healthy, but first, discuss the fill-in-the-blank questions from days 1–5 and the action steps listed at the end of day 5 in session 3. *(Leader: discuss session 3 questions before proceeding.)*

Next read the fourth chapter of *7 Steps to Get Off Sugar and Carbo-hydrates*, Step 4: Purchase Healthy Foods and an Anti-Candida Cleanse. Each member can read one paragraph or section out loud to the group. Whatever portion of the chapter you are not able to finish should be assigned as homework. Ask the following questions after reading each section.

Healthy Foods to Purchase

Now that you've removed all the unhealthy food from your kitchen, it is time to stock up with healthy choices. You can purchase a vast number of organic vegetables, fruits, nuts, seeds, whole grains (organic oats, brown rice, quinoa, barley), beans, fish, and meat. Each is unique in its flavor and amount of nutrients. Therefore, we should vary the types of foods we eat so we consume a variety of vitamins and minerals.

Our Creator gave us an abundant number of vegetables to choose from:

- artichoke
- asparagus
- avocado (technically a fruit)
- beans: azuki, black, broad, green, kidney, lima, mung, navy, pinto, snow, soy, sugar snap
- beet
- broccoli
- brussel sprout
- bok choy
- cabbage: kohlrabi
- carrot
- cauliflower
- celery
- collard greens
- corn
- daikon
- eggplant
- kale
- lentils
- lettuce: arugula, buttercrunch, endive, iceburg, oak leaf, mache, mesclun, romaine, radicchio, watercress
- mustard greens
- okra
- onions: chives, garlic, leek, shallot, scallion
- peas: black-eyed, chickpeas (garbanzo), split
- peppers: bell, chili (jalapeno, habanero, cayenne)

- potatoes: red, white, sweet
- pumpkin
- radish
- rhubarb
- rutabaga
- spinach
- squash: acorn, butternut, patty pan, spaghetti, zucchini
- swiss chard
- tomato (technically a fruit)
- turnip greens

Do you tend to eat the same type of vegetables over and over? If yes, what new vegetable can you try? (Choose from the list above.)

_____

Seeds contain trace minerals. The following list of seeds will help you incorporate these micronutrients into your diet:

- chia
- flax
- hemp
- poppy
- pumpkin
- sesame
- sunflower

Do you include seeds into your diet? If yes, which ones? If not, what will you choose to add? (Choose from the list above.)

_____

Nuts are an excellent source of protein. Purchase raw nuts rather than roasted, salted, or sugar coated ones because they contain more nutrition in their natural form. God created numerous varieties of nuts to choose from:

- almond
- brazil
- cashew
- chestnut
- hazelnut
- macadamia
- pecan
- pistachio
- pine
- walnut

Which nuts do you like and which ones will you add to your diet? What new nut can you try? (Choose from the selection above.)

_____

. . .

Which variety of nut grows in your region of the country? Could you visit a nut orchard near you and purchase fresh nuts? (I store local pecans in my freezer for months.)

Healthy Eating Guidelines

Chapter 4 and appendix 5 of *7 Steps to Get Off Sugar and Carbohydrates* provide healthy eating guidelines to keep you on track with your new food regimen. You can obtain a printable version of the appendices at SusanUNeal.com/appendix.

Which healthy eating guideline do you think would be most difficult to integrate and why?

Is the 80/20-percent rule practical for you? If yes, why? If not, why not?

Healthy Substitutes to Purchase

Do you currently use any sugar, dairy, or pasta substitutes listed in chapter 4? If yes, which ones? If not, which one will you commit to try?

_____

Have you tried spaghetti squash or spiralized zucchini as a pasta substitute? If yes, did you like it? How did you use it?

_____

Water

Calculate the number of eight ounce glasses of water you should drink per day based on your weight. (Pounds/2 = # ounces; # ounces/8 ounces (1 cup) = # cups.)

_____

Do you drink the recommended amount of water per day? If not, how can you increase your water intake?

_____

Foods that Cause Inflammation

Did you know the two most inflammation-causing foods are sugar and wheat? What did you learn about these two foods from the book so far? What difference does this information make in your personal food choices?

. . .

_____

_____

Gut Health

Have you ever taken an antibiotic? If yes, afterward, did you take a probiotic or cultured food product to replace the beneficial bacteria in your gut? If you didn't replenish your gut flora, you are more likely to have a candida infection.

Do you regularly take a probiotic supplement? If yes, does it contain ten different strains of beneficial bacteria? List several places you can search to find the right kind of probiotic.

_____

Weekly Menu Planning

Is menu planning enjoyable for you? If not, is there someone in your family or a friend you could do your menu planning with?

_____

Check out menus, recipes, and corresponding grocery lists on Susan-UNeal.com/healthy-living-blog.

. . .

Uncooperative Family Member

Some of you may encounter family members who are not willing to change their eating habits. I faced this in my home. We can't change their attitudes, but we are in control of how we react to them. An attitude of grace and understanding toward their food choices is best. Accommodating their food selection decreases contention.

You are making these changes to improve your health and weight. Everyone in your home will benefit from your improvement because you will have more energy to upkeep the home.

For me, it was necessary to improve my diet to heal my body. However, to accommodate everyone I provided several vegetable and grain choices at mealtime. That way, everyone could choose which food item they felt was best for them.

I cooked two or three vegetables instead of one, and two grains. My family members preferred the pasta or white rice, but I made spaghetti squash or quinoa for me. One of my daughters tried the spaghetti squash and liked it. Thereafter, she chose to eat the squash instead of the pasta. Ultimately, our family transitioned to eating brown rice instead of white. It was a slow process, but when they saw how my health improved, their uncooperativeness softened.

Do you have someone in your home who may be uncooperative? If yes, who? How do you think you could persuade them to try some new dishes?

_____

_____

Ask your Bible study group and prayer partner to pray for the inflexible situations you may encounter and how you should handle them.

. . .

Journal

Are you using your *Healthy Living Journal*? If yes, what revelations did you figure out about your lifestyle choices and your health?

_____

Conclusion

A support system is essential when making these lifestyle changes. This study group is an integral part of that system. Encourage and support each other along the journey to improve your health and be sure to pray for each other.

As a group, decide whether you want to read the fifth chapter of *7 Steps to Get Off Sugar and Carbohydrates*, Step 5: Plan for the Start Date, on your own or during session 5.

DAY 1: MENU PLANNING

Last week you tackled the monumental task of cleaning out the pantry, refrigerator, and freezer. This week you should take a trip to the grocery store and purchase healthy foods to replace the ones you disposed of. But first, you need to plan your menu and corresponding grocery list.

To ease the task of menu planning, I created a standard grocery list for the store I used. To create this list, initially I walked through the store and either wrote or dictated into my smartphone notes app the items I normally purchased on each grocery aisle. For example, I would start in the back of the store in the refrigerated section and would include eggs, butter, and coconut milk on the list for that aisle. Then I proceeded to the next aisle: cleaning supplies and paper products. I listed toilet paper, napkins, paper towels, paper plates, etc. And so on, until I compiled a master grocery list. At home, I typed out this list based on each grocery store aisle and the products I usually purchased. It took work to create this list, but it streamlined my grocery store planning for years.

Each week I printed a fresh new grocery list and my family knew that if we ran out of an item, they were supposed to circle it on the list or write it out. I made a rule to guide us—if it wasn't on the list, it didn't get purchased. I put the responsibility on them, not all on me.

Planning my weekly menu takes about an hour, and I usually do this on Sunday. I list what I plan to cook for breakfast, lunch, dinner, and snack for every day of the week. As I choose a recipe, I put the ingredients I need on my corresponding grocery list. For years, as my children grew up, I posted on their chalkboard what the menu was for every day of the week. Everyone in the family knew what I would be serving.

I cooked on Sunday and Monday and listed leftovers (from Sunday) to be served on Tuesday. Wednesday we all ate at church, and Thursday I served leftovers from Monday. To liven up a leftover, I would cook one new item (such as a vegetable) to be served with the previous meal, and this new item gave the meal new interest. Two nights of cooking took care of four meals.

Every week I made a large, fresh, raw salad (broccoli salad, beet salad, cole slaw, salad with lettuce) and I ate that for my lunch throughout the week. For my children's lunch boxes, I tried to include one fresh fruit and vegetable each day.

After you create your menu and corresponding grocery list (subscribe to SusanUNeal.com/healthy-living-blog for menus and lists), hit the grocery store or local farmer's market. Once your groceries are put away, start cooking healthy homemade meals. Your body will appreciate your planning and food preparation, and being prepared will keep you from making unhealthy impulsive choices when you grocery shop.

DAY 2: PURCHASE AN ANTI-CANDIDA CLEANSE

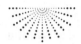

Candida Albicans is a form of yeast and causes the most common type of yeast infections. If you tested positive for the Candida spit test, described in step 2 of *7 Steps to Get Off Sugar and Carbohydrates*, purchase an anti-Candida cleanse. Cleanses are available at health food stores and online. An attendant at the health food store can tell you the best cleanse they carry.

If you had a negative Candida spit test, there is no need to purchase or take the anti-Candida cleanse. In fact, you may not need a daily probiotic either. However, if you take antibiotics in the future, be sure to follow-up with a bottle of a probiotic that contains ten strains of beneficial microorganisms.

If you need to take the cleanse, wait to take it until session 5 when specific instructions are provided. In the meantime, take a probiotic supplement every morning. I take mine as I drink two glasses of filtered water before breakfast.

Probiotics enhance the balance of the beneficial microorganisms with the bad (Candida) in our gastrointestinal (GI) systems. Similarly, godly habits such as attending church; fellowshipping with other Christians; and reading and studying the Word of God through daily devotions, Bible study, or Sunday school enhance our spiritual life and decrease the harmful practices of sin.

When we get out of the habit of attending church, and we don't take time for a daily devotions, it's like we're not taking our probiotic and the Candida, or sin, overgrows. Passages in the Old Testament compare yeast to sin or evil (Exodus 12:15; Leviticus 2:11). Jesus told us to beware of the yeast (sin) of the Pharisees (Matthew 16:6), and Paul wrote, "Don't you realize that this sin is like a little yeast that spreads through the whole batch of dough? Get rid of the old 'yeast' . . . Then you will be like a fresh batch of dough made without yeast, which is what you really are" (1 Corinthians 5:6–7).

All we need is a little bit of sin or yeast (Candida) to creep into our lives, and it grows exponentially. Only as a teaspoon of yeast makes the whole batch of dough rise, likewise, a little sin mushrooms in a person's life. The progression of sinning or Candidiasis (Candida infection from a Candida fungus) occurs in our spiritual life and physical bodies without us even realizing it. So beware of the yeast.

Spiritually, sin may begin as a lie or deception that propagates because we need to hide it. Pretty soon one lie turns into ten, but you did not mean for it to. Physically, antibiotics are like that first lie or deception; they kill the beneficial microorganisms in the gut, so Candida has a chance to flourish, taking over the digestive tract. The more often we take antibiotics, the more this unhealthy process continues.

Candida can grow roots into the lining of the GI tract. The fungal overgrowth creates openings in the bowel walls, which is known as a leaky gut. These holes allow harmful microorganisms to enter the bloodstream. Our bodies don't recognize these particles. Therefore, our immune system creates antibodies, which cause food allergies and autoimmune diseases to develop.[1] An overgrowth of Candida also causes our abdomen to become distended.

Similarly, a little sin can ruin a whole life. Our sin may start with one occurrence, but when we continue to lie or deceive others, we quench the Holy Spirit. The Holy Spirit's guidance in our life is subtle. Many times we don't recognize God's nudging through his Spirit.

In 1 Kings 19:12 God's voice is described as a "gentle whisper," so his voice can be hard to identify. Therefore, we need to spend time with him in order to recognize his voice. We learn to hear him as we pray and meditate. Quiet your mind and spend a few minutes of uninterrupted time with the Lord listening for him. The Lord also speaks to us through Scripture. The more we read passages from the Bible and devotions, the more we become aware of his supernatural presence within us.

Part of the Holy Spirit's job is to convict us of sin. However, if we don't listen to the initial prompting of the Spirit, we become less sensitive to its urging, and sin (or yeast) escalates. When we recognize the Spirit's guidance in our life, we choose whether to obey or resist it. If we decide to ignore it, we have less of God's power and may find ourselves battling temptations on our own. Therefore, we are more likely to yield to our fleshly desires.

When sin or Candida spreads out of control, it acts like a parasite sucking the life and energy out of you. Candida feeds on carbs, which is why you crave them. It is like a monster growing inside of you, craving sugar, and it is hard to fight its never-ending appetite. Likewise, when you are used to succumbing to temptation, it becomes easier to sin.

To be wholly healthy, we need to get both our gastrointestinal system and spiritual life into balance. Once you've completed the anti-Candida cleanse and take a daily probiotic, you will be well on your way to balancing that area of your body. Probiotics are like the godly habits you should routinely perform to keep your spiritual life in balance.

To kill the yeast we take an anti-Candida cleanse. But how do we master sin? We repent at the moment we realize we sinned. We shouldn't wait until the next day or when we have time to spend with God. Instead, at the moment we become aware that we sinned, we should ask for forgiveness.

. . .

Now take a moment, and close your eyes. Ask God to reveal any hidden sin in your life. Meditate and see if God's brings any thoughts to the forefront of your mind. What do you need to ask him to forgive?

We stop the sin (yeast) before it grows if we repent immediately. The next time you sin, ask Jesus to forgive you right after you realized you sinned. If you are genuinely sorry and try your best to turn away from that sin, he will forgive you. It takes effort to balance the physical and spiritual dimensions of your life, but with the help of Christ, you can do it!

What obstacles have you experienced in dealing with both Candida and sin? What steps will you take to overcome these obstacles so neither will continue to grow?

DAY 3: DANIEL'S RESOLVE

The first obstacle to overcome in eliminating sugar and carbohydrates is to *decide*—decide to improve your eating habits. This is the first step in our seven-step plan. Once you've decided to make this lifestyle change, with the help of Christ, you can succeed. Along the way, you may need to return to that original decision and recommit to it as situations (like vacations, weddings, and parties) or temptations challenge your original decision. Continually stand firm in that original decision even when you falter from time to time.

The biblical character Daniel exemplified decision making. He chose to avoid the unhealthy food choices of the Babylonians. "Daniel made up his mind not to harm himself by eating the king's rich food and drinking the king's wine. So he asked the chief-of-staff for permission not to harm himself in this way" (Daniel 1:8, GW).

In this verse "made up his mind" means "having reached a decision; firmly resolved; showing determination." Firmly resolving to change your eating habits is half your battle. Once you make up your mind to do something, you can achieve amazing results, particularly if you ask for God's help.

. . .

Did you "made up your mind" to change your eating habits? If yes, how did you come to this decision? For example, are you in poor health or tired of being overweight?

What type of resolve did you experience in the last four weeks to maintain your commitment? What helped you stick to it?

With a firm decision to improve your health, you can replace negative habits with positive ones. For example, if you substitute several soft drinks a day with water, think of the changes that would occur in your body over the course of a year. You would lose weight, experience more energy, and be in better health physiologically, simply by making this one change. As you improve your eating habits, you will achieve abundant results and reclaim the health Jesus wants you to experience.

DAY 4: DANIEL'S VEGETABLES

After Daniel resolved not to eat the king's food, he had to get special permission from his superior.

> Daniel said to the supervisor, "Please test us for ten days. Give us only vegetables to eat and water to drink. Then compare us to the young men who are eating the king's rich food. Decide how to treat us on the basis of how we look."
> The supervisor listened to them about this matter and tested them for ten days. After ten days they looked healthier and stronger than the young men who had been eating the king's rich food.
>
> Daniel 1:11–15 (GW)

Daniel convinced his supervisor to let his friends and him eat vegetables. The results were astonishing as they were "healthier and stronger" than their counterparts.

God created over one hundred vegetables, so Daniel probably had a large variety of food options provided to him. Each vegetable contains various types of nutrients essential for proper growth and performance. Bread, processed foods, and sugar-laden products do not give the body the vitamins and minerals it needs to recreate properly functioning cells.

Today, many people eat food packaged in boxes and bags because it is convenient. Unfortunately, the nutrients our Creator put into fruits, vegetables, and grains get stripped away as these packaged foods are processed, so they can be stored on the grocery shelves for months, if not years. Therefore, we starve ourselves of essential nutrients the body requires to be healthy. No wonder over half of Americans live with a chronic illness. Apparently, we are not eating the foods God designed, but the foods manufacturers create for their profit.

We see from Daniel's experiment that produce grown from seeds (vegetables) made him healthier and stronger than his counterparts. We should follow Daniel's lead and increase our consumption of vegetables, grains (except hybridized wheat or Roundup Ready corn and grains), nuts, seeds, and fruit; and stop eating processed foods that have little or no nutritional value.

Daniel served numerous kings, including King Cyrus of Persia. Therefore, Daniel lived over eighty years and possible close to ninety. Have you ever thought about the long lifespan mankind experienced before the flood? Noah was 950 years old when he died (Genesis 7:6; 9:28). Whereas, Moses only lived 120 years (Deuteronomy 34:7), and King David died at 70 years of age (2 Samuel 5:4). Therefore, during the years following the flood the Bible records a progressive decline in man's lifespan.

What do you think may have caused this progressive decline in lifespan?

. . .

I believe it is due to the introduction of meat into the human diet. After the flood God told Noah:

> "All the animals of the earth, all the birds of the sky, all the small animals that scurry along the ground, and all the fish in the sea will look on you with fear and terror. I have placed them in your power. I have given them to you for food, just as I have given you grain and vegetables."
>
> Genesis 9:2–3

Prior to the flood mankind was a vegetarian. What does eating meat have to do with longevity? The fat in meat clogs arteries with plaque. Atherosclerosis (clogged arteries) causes heart disease and strokes (two of the top five leading causes of death in the US).[2]

At age eighty-four, my mother suffered a stroke that caused dementia, so I researched how to decrease my chance of a stroke. I could significantly reduce my risk of a stroke and heart disease by becoming a vegetarian.[3] Therefore, I decreased my consumption of meat and increased healthier protein alternatives.

Nuts, beans, and seeds are excellent sources of protein, and fish is a healthier type of meat because most types contain omega-3 fatty acids. Every week, I prepare a few meals with one of these meat substitutes as the primary protein source. I may serve fish one night, beans another, and nuts on my salad for a third. I still cook poultry and beef, but I serve it less frequently. However, I avoid pork because if this meat is undercooked, and the animal is infected with the Trichinella worm, a person could become infected with trichinosis.

Another protein alternative is whole grain quinoa, which contains ten grams of protein in one cup (cooked). I sauté fresh vegetables and combine them with quinoa for a satisfying meal that takes only twenty minutes to prepare. (Quinoa recipes are included in appendix 4 of *7 Steps to Get Off Sugar and Carbohydrates*.) Countless vegetable combinations can be created.

God gave us a vast variety of vegetables to tantalize our palates and provide what our bodies need. Avoid falling into the modern-day trap of eating processed foods; instead, eat the foods our Creator provided. Evaluate everything you eat: did God create this food or did a manufacturer? Your body will thank you when you eat the foods God intended rather than what manufacturers fabricated.

DAY 5: CHANGE YOUR MIND-SET

During this lifestyle change you will experience good and bad days. On the hard days, you might believe all sorts of lies. Therefore, your thought life could be an obstacle to making changes to improve your health. The challenge is not to let yourself become defeated on the bad days, but focus on your victories.

Our enemy can attack us through our mind because we are not fighting against flesh and blood. Ignore the lies of the enemy that say you failed. Instead, fight the unseen forces with God's weapons, as Paul tells us to do in 2 Corinthians 10:3–4: "We are human, but we don't wage war as humans do. We use God's mighty weapons, not worldly weapons, to knock down the strongholds of human reasoning and to destroy false arguments."

God's weapons include prayer, praise, and the sword of the Spirit (speaking Bible verses out loud).[4] Use them to destroy the false arguments placed in your mind through doubts, fears, and a defeated outlook.

1. Prayer: On the tough days, pray and ask Jesus to intercede for you. He is our high priest.

2. Praise: Lift your arms while listening to praise music. Demonic forces can't stand to be around a person who is praising the Lord.
3. Sword of the Spirit: Memorize and utilize your strategic Bible verse. Scripture is the sword God gave you. Use it.

Second Corinthians 10:5 teaches us how to fight the enemy's false arguments: "We demolish arguments and every pretension that sets itself up against the knowledge of God, and we take captive every thought to make it obedient to Christ" (NIV). I used the strategy from this verse to train my mind to bring every negative thought to Jesus and asked him to remove it. This tactic works. Next time you feel defeated, tell Christ how you feel and ask him to help you replace deceptive thoughts with truthful ones.

You can renew your mind (replace negative thoughts with positive ones) through the Word of God. To do this read passages of scripture and attend church, Sunday school, or a Bible study. Spend regular quality time with the Lord and pray, because the strength of your spiritual life is dependent upon it.

Choose to focus on positive thoughts, not the ones the enemy wants you to dwell on. However, renewing the mind takes place a little at a time. You have to consciously choose the right thoughts and reject the wrong ones. When you can't seem to brush off the enemy's condemnation, use your weapons of prayer, praise, and God's Word to defeat him.

The mind needs to be renewed and follow the Spirit of God, not the flesh.[6] Capture the enemy's deceptive lies so they do not defeat you. Recognize what you're thinking and choose your thoughts carefully, because Proverbs 23:7 tells us, "For as he thinks in his heart, so *is* he" (NKJV). Even on the days you count as a loss, you can celebrate at least one small victory to keep from feeling defeated. Focus on that success and write it in your journal. Meditate on your Bible verse. Change your mind-set!

When you feel discouraged or condemned, examine your thought life. Changing your thinking will set you free. Emphasize the progress you've made, not the failures. Stop your mind from taking you down the path of defeat. Instead, focus on one victory where you were strong and recognize you can be strong in other areas as well. This is the truth. Better yet, turn an unhealthy behavior into a new healthy living habit you incorporate into your life. The *Healthy Living Journal* contains a New Healthy Living Habits section for you to record your new routines.

Session 4 Action Steps

1. Read the fourth chapter of *7 Steps to Get Off Sugar and Carbohydrates*, Step 4: Purchase Healthy Foods and an Anti-Candida Cleanse.
2. Prepare your menu and corresponding grocery list.
3. Purchase healthy foods.
4. If needed, buy an anti-Candida cleanse.
5. Take a probiotic supplement.
6. Do not purchase or eat processed foods out of boxes and bags.
7. Replace some servings of meat with alternative protein sources.
8. Train yourself to bring every negative thought to Jesus and ask him to remove it from your mind.
9. On bad days, focus on your victories not your failures.
10. Record new healthy living habits in your journal.

PART V

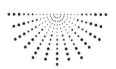

SESSION 5: IMPLEMENT THE PLAN

For the past four weeks you prepared so you would be ready to implement the physical and spiritual plans for getting off sugar and carbs. You:

- *decided* (step 1) to make a lifestyle change and improve your health.
- *acquired knowledge* (step 2) about changing your eating habits and identified your support system.
- *cleaned out* (step 3) your pantry, refrigerator, and emotions.
- *purchased* (step 4) groceries, based on the healthy eating guidelines, and an anti-Candida cleanse.

This week you will implement what you learned, but first, please discuss the fill-in-the-blank questions and action steps from the end of session 4. (*Leader: discuss session 4 questions before proceeding.*)

Read the fifth chapter of *7 Steps to Get Off Sugar and Carbohydrates*, Step 5: Plan for the Start Date. Each member can read one paragraph or section out loud to the group. Whatever portion of the chapter you are not able to finish should be assigned as homework. Ask the following questions after reading each section.

Seven-Day Eating Plan

Do you consume the recommended amount of water? If you do not consume the suggested amount of water, do you think the recommendation of drinking two glasses of water before each meal will help? How can you plan to commit to this step?

Have you started taking a daily probiotic? If yes, have you noticed that you experience more energy?

What will be most difficult for you: eliminating wheat or high-sugar foods (> 10 grams of sugar per serving)? Why?

Are you going to take an anti-Candida cleanse? If yes, when do you plan to start?

Do you routinely exercise? If yes, what type of activity do you perform? Do you enjoy this type of exercise?

If you do not routinely exercise, what type of workout do you enjoy? How can you incorporate an enjoyable form of activity into your life?

Binding the Strong Man in Your Life

Discuss how an addiction can be a "strong man" in your life.

Please write the Five-Step Binding the Strong Man Plan below. The steps are listed in appendix 8 in *7 Steps to Get Off Sugar and Carbohydrates*.

. . .

Did you select your key Bible verse, yet? If yes, please write it below. If not, choose one and write it here.

Which do you think will be more difficult, implementing the physical Seven-Day Eating Plan or the spiritual Five-Step Binding the Strong Man Plan? Why?

Conclusion

This chapter outlines the strategy for getting off sugar and carbs. Weaning yourself off these products is more difficult than most people think, which is why many are not successful. However, when you use the spiritual plan and access God's power, instead of relying on your own, you can succeed. Addressing the spiritual component of our being cuts through the unseen forces acting against us. May God bless your endeavor to improve your lifestyle.

DAY 1: IMPLEMENT THE SEVEN-DAY EATING PLAN

You acquired knowledge about changing your eating habits, selected your support system, cleaned out the pantry, and purchased groceries based on the healthy eating guidelines. Now it is time to implement the physical plan to wean yourself off carbs and sugar.

If you haven't done so already, obtain a printable version of the appendices in *7 Steps to Get Off Sugar and Carbohydrates* by going to SusanUNeal.com/appendix. Print out Appendix 6: Seven-Day Eating Plan and post it on your refrigerator, so it is readily available.

Write down when you will begin implementing the seven-day plan.

_____

Let your family and prayer partner know the date you will start the plan. You need the support of family and friends when changing your lifestyle. Follow the steps below (on the date you chose) to begin.

. . .

Seven-Day Eating Plan

Day 1 (Start on Wednesday)

1. Consume Water
Drink up to two cups of coffee or tea per day, but no more. The only other beverage you should drink is filtered water. I use a filter on my refrigerator water dispenser and a water filter on a pitcher. Before breakfast drink two glasses of water, two before lunch, two midafternoon, and two more before dinner. Do not drink during meals and do not drink anything after dinner. Drink up to ten minutes before eating. Keep track of how much you drink in the Water Tracker chart in your *Healthy Living Journal*.

2. Take a Probiotic
Begin taking a probiotic every day. Make sure it contains at least ten different strains of beneficial bacteria. Record when you take a probiotic in the Well-Being Chart in the *Healthy Living Journal*.

3. Stop Eating High-Sugar Foods
Stop eating anything containing more than 10 grams of sugar per serving. Check labels for the number of grams of sugar per serving size.

Day 2

1. Eliminate Wheat
Do not eat anything containing wheat. No more bagels, toast, pancakes, biscuits, pasta, pretzels, crackers, cookies, cake, or pie. Eliminating wheat is like going off a drug. Be aware that you may experience the following symptoms for a few days: irritability, foggy brain, and fatigue. You might even feel fluish. However, within a week

your symptoms will subside. After this, avoid eating wheat or consuming foods with more than 10 grams of sugar in one serving, or your addiction will start all over again. (Ugh.)

Day 3

1. Eliminate Processed Foods
Do not eat processed foods from boxes and bags.

2. Implement Healthy Eating Guidelines
Make 50 percent of your food fresh and raw. By raw, I mean uncooked foods such as salads, fruit, and uncooked vegetables. Follow the Healthy Eating Guidelines provided in appendix 5 of *7 Steps to Get Off Sugar and Carbohydrates.*

Days 4 and 5 (Saturday and Sunday)

Continue to implement all the steps listed on day one through three as you proceed.

1. Rest
Focus on you. Rest, read, pray, and ask God to help you succeed.

2. Use the Sword of the Spirit
Now is the time to fight the thief Jesus spoke of in John 10:10, for Satan wants you to fail: "The thief's purpose is to steal, kill and destroy. My purpose is to give life in all its fullness" (John 10:10 TLB). Fight the thief with the sword of the Spirit—the Word of God. Have you written your key verse on index cards or put it on the notes app on your smartphone? Every time you get the urge to go back to your old eating habits, speak the verse out loud to cut any demonic influences out of your life. Address your spiritual nature as well as your physical.

Day 6

1. Start the Anti-Candida Cleanse

Now let's kill the bug in your gut—Candida. If you tested positive for
the Candida test in step 1, start the anti-Candida cleanse you
purchased in step 4. If you are not ready to begin this step because
you are still experiencing symptoms of withdrawal (headache, exhaustion, irritability, mental fogginess, fluish symptoms), wait a few days
until you feel better.

Read the instructions on the cleanse package for how to administer it. Initially, I recommend taking the cleanse every other day for
the first week to minimize lethargy and headaches. You will feel awful
if the dead Candida is not quickly expelled from your colon. To avoid
becoming constipated, drink plenty of water. During the second
week, begin taking the Candida cleanse every day as recommended.

Prevent a headache by increasing the fiber in your diet through a
fiber supplement (which usually comes with your Candida cleanse),
water, and raw fruits and vegetables. The first three days you are on
the cleanse, you may not feel well, but after a week you will begin to
feel better than you have in a long time. You are just about to regain
the life Jesus wants you to experience—one that is abundant and full.

Day 7

1. Get Up and Exercise

If you are still feeling the symptoms of withdrawal, be gentle with
yourself by performing a simple form of exercise such as walking or
yoga. It doesn't matter what type of activity you do, as long as you do
it. Walking, jumping rope, lifting weights, or taking a group fitness
class like Pilates or water aerobics are a few examples of exercise.
When you begin to feel better, try to exercise for twenty minutes

three times a week. Record the activity you perform in the Fitness or Steps Tracker in the *Healthy Living Journal*.

In addition to physical movement, mindfulness exercises such as yoga and meditation train a person to pay attention to cravings without reacting to them. The idea is to ride out the wave of intense desire. As a person becomes more mindful, she notices why she wants to indulge. Meditation quiets the part of the brain that can lead to a loop of obsession.[1] Check out my website at ChristianYoga.com for products that can increase your mindfulness.

Day 8 and Beyond

You are well on your way to changing your lifestyle, but more than that, you will change your life for the better. Your health, mood, and energy level will improve. Each week you will lose unhealthy weight, and the body God gave you will heal itself of many ailments. As your body heals from disease, you will be able to reduce or eliminate medications because you no longer suffer from the symptoms these medications treated. However, *before stopping any prescription medication, be sure to consult with your physician.*

Increased vitality will allow you to experience activities you were unable to enjoy before. Overall your well-being and emotional countenance will be revitalized. You are in the process of getting your life back, the one the Lord wants you to enjoy to its fullest.

DAY 2: IMPLEMENT THE FIVE-STEP BINDING THE STRONG MAN PLAN

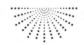

The Seven-Step Eating Plan is effective because it addresses both our physical bodies and spiritual nature. In the Five-Step Binding the Strong Man Plan, a person does not rely on his or her willpower but accesses God's mighty power instead. Therefore, it is instrumental to begin the following spiritual plan when you perform the Seven-Step Eating Plan. Unsheathe the spiritual weapons God gave you and kick the evil spiritual forces right out of your life.

First, print a copy of appendix 8 from *7 Steps to Get Off Sugar and Carbohydrates* by going to SusanUNeal.com/appendix. Post the Five-Step Binding the Strong Man Plan on your refrigerator, so it is easily accessible.

Every morning implement the five-step plan listed below. Make this a daily priority as you implement the eating plan. Also, listen to worship music as you get ready for the day, and be sure to praise God. This will get the dopamine (a feel-good neurohormone) flowing and make unseen demonic forces flee.

Five-Step Binding the Strong Man Plan
   1. Name what controls you.

Name the thing controlling you—food addiction, anxiety, eating disorder, depression, etc.—whatever it may be, and declare (out loud) Jesus Christ is your Lord in its place![2]

Stand up to the evil spirit who brought bondage into your life by saying, "Evil spirit, you won't lord over me or entice me through (insert your addiction) anymore. Jesus is my Lord!" A person obtains spiritual power and authority through Christ. Declare that the spiritual powers of darkness will not have lordship over your life. They will not rule you, govern your behavior, capture your thought life, or lead you into temptation and sin because "the one who is in you is greater than the one who is in the world" (1 John 4:4 NIV).

> For when Satan, strong and fully armed, guards his palace, it is safe—
> until someone stronger and better armed attacks and overcomes him
> and strips him of his weapons and carries off his belongings.
>
> Luke 11:21–22 (TLB)

Get ready, for *you are capable of evicting the addiction strong man in your life*. If you accepted Jesus as your Lord and Savior (see appendix 7 in *7 Steps to Get Off Sugar and Carbohydrates*), the Holy Spirit lives within you and the Spirit is stronger than Satan. Day after day, declare out loud that Jesus reigns as the Lord of your life—not your addiction.

2. Submit yourself completely to God.

> Submit yourself to God, resist the devil and he will flee from you.
>
> James 4:7 (NIV)

There is a secret to resisting the devil—you must first submit yourself to God. How in the world do you do that? In my experience, you no longer do your will but the Lord's will by submitting your life to him. For me, it was not without a fight.

If you are a food addict, after binging, ask God to forgive you and help you not to binge again. Document the experience in the *Healthy Living Journal*'s Binge Eating Tracker. Once you ask for forgiveness, he chooses not to remember your sins, as indicated in Hebrews 8:12: "And I will be merciful to them in their wrongdoings, and I will remember their sins no more" (TLB). Don't fret over a stumble. Get up and try again using this Five-Step Binding the Strong Man Plan.

3. Use the name of Jesus.

Jesus told his disciples, "Look, I have given you authority over all the power of the enemy" (Luke 10:19). If you are a disciple of Jesus, you can accept the authority he gave you.

In the book of Acts, the apostles healed and worked miracles in the name of Jesus. Use Jesus's name as Peter did in Acts 3:6: "In the name of Jesus Christ of Nazareth, walk" (TLB). Using the name of Jesus is key to binding the strong man because then you operate under Jesus's authority.

Picture a person tied in ropes. That's the way a spiritual strong man afflicts his victim. However, if you declare Jesus is Lord over your life, not the strong man (addiction), and use Jesus's name, you are under his authority. Then the spiritual ropes, tied around you by the evil spirit, loosen and fall off. Next comes the moment to take action by tying the strong man through binding him with the Word of God.

4. Use the Word of God.

For when Satan, strong and fully armed, guards his palace, it is safe— until someone stronger and better armed attacks and overcomes him and strips him of his weapons and carries off his belongings.

Luke 11:21–22 TLB

The Holy Spirit inside of you is stronger than Satan and his demons. By using the name of Jesus, you are not only under his authority but you also speak with his authority. You are much better armed than Satan. Now is the time to stand up to him, strip him of his weapons, and kick him out of your life through the Word of God! Say to the strong man, "In the name of Jesus, you won't oppress me anymore. I bind your power in the name of Jesus and by the Word of God."

Use the specific scripture you chose to bind the strong man every time he tempts you. Have you memorized your verse yet? It is your spiritual sword. If you do not use it you may not succeed in this fight to recover your health.

Luke 11:22 states the strong man was stripped of his weapons and his belongings were carried off. Matthew 12:29 asserts that when Satan was bound, his demons could be cast out. After you tie up the strong man with the Word of God—ignore him. He will try to hobble after you because he doesn't give up easily. If he did, he wouldn't be a strong man. The next time you are tempted, you're facing a critical moment. When you give him (the spirit of addiction) your attention by drinking or eating sugary foods, binging, etc. you are, in effect, untying the strong man.

5. Praise God and practice gratitude.

When you praise God and thank him for his blessings, the strong man won't hang around. Don't be satisfied with binding the strong man and walking away—punish him.

Fill your mind, heart, and body with the Spirit of God by putting the right things in your spirit. Listen to praise music; read the Bible and pray; memorize scripture; attend church, Sunday school, or a Bible study. Also start doing more to help others. Performing acts of service and helping others fills your heart with honorable feelings and humility. Every day write in your journal about all you can praise God for and thank him.

Beat the strong man by declaring Bible verses out loud. Stomp him into the ground by singing praises to the Lord. The devil can't stand to be around someone who worships the Lord.

Become God's warrior by using his mighty weapons. Paul advises, "It is true that I am an ordinary, weak human being, but I don't use human plans and methods to win my battles. I use God's mighty weapons, not those made by men, to knock down the devil's strongholds" (2 Corinthians 10:3–4 TLB). Get ready to knock out and tie up the strong man of addiction in your life. You are God's mighty conqueror!

DAY 3: USE THE LORD'S POWER

We started the step-by-step eating plan and daily five-step spiritual plan. Next we will learn more about the unseen spiritual forces that exist in this world, as we are not fighting against flesh and blood (other people) but evil forces of Satan.

A final word: Be strong in the Lord and in his mighty power. Put on all of God's armor so that you will be able to stand firm against all strategies of the devil. For we are not fighting against flesh-and-blood enemies, but against evil rulers and authorities of the unseen world, against mighty powers in this dark world, and against evil spirits in the heavenly places.

Ephesians 6:10–12

Who are the evil rulers and authorities, mighty powers, and evil spirits described in this verse? These spiritual beings are Satan's army. Satan does not like believers (people who accepted Christ as their

Savior) because they have been snatched from his kingdom and now are part of God's kingdom.[3] Therefore, he uses his army to harm us.

Ephesians 6 tells us that the devil uses *strategies*, which means "crafty schemes with the intent to deceive." Satan understands mankind's fleshly desires and tendency toward sin, so he uses every opportunity to take advantage of these weaknesses. One of them being our appetites. Every time we eat, we choose between God's provision and man's perversion.

While food doesn't seem like it would be a big deal in the spiritual battle, it is an instrument of bondage and destruction the enemy uses. It's not really about the food but control. Satan knows how he can distract us from living the life the Lord intended. Food is a tool Satan uses, a button he pushes, to get our bodies and thoughts out of alignment with God and make us think negatively about ourselves. Therefore, our inappropriate food choices affect our relationship with the Lord and impact his kingdom.

When you are unhealthy you cannot fulfill the mission God intended for you. Jesus told us "the thief's purpose is to steal, kill, and destroy" (John 10:10). What better way to harm us than through health problems caused by unhealthy eating habits? Shortening our lifespan is the enemy's perfect scheme. He is doing a great job of it too, since over half of Americans have a chronic disease and 40 percent suffer from obesity.

Are you fulfilling the mission the Lord gave to you? If not, is your health or stamina holding you back?

Whether you like it or not, you are in a battle to get your health and weight back to normal. To help you with temptation print the list of Food Addiction Battle Strategies from appendix 10 of *7 Steps to Get*

Off Sugar and Carbohydrates, and use these strategies if and when you stumble.

On your quest to improve your well-being you need to prepare to engage in spiritual warfare. Just as Daniel resolved not to eat the king's food, you must stand firm in your decision to continue this quest no matter how many times you slip up.

Open your eyes to the spirit realm and become more mindful of situations that might have a spiritual alignment. When you understand who you fight against, you can feel the evil forces compelling you to eat delicious foods you know are not good for you.

Do you experience this type of temptation? If yes, when is it most likely to occur?

_____

Paul explains we are to "be strong in the Lord and in his mighty power." In whose power? The Lord's. When we use Jesus's power, through the Holy Spirit, we become strong and able to do something we could not do on our own. Through his power we are capable of defeating the enemy.

How do we access God's power? Through abiding in Christ and following the Holy Spirit's guidance in our life. Talk to Jesus throughout the day and ask him to support you with your daily challenges. Listen to the Spirit's quiet guidance. Tapping into his power will help you make better choices and persevere when tempted.

We live in an indulgent culture that makes it challenging to avoid delectable treats such as donuts, birthday cake, and unhealthy foods at potluck dinners. If we live for God, we must purposefully resist worldly temptations. We can't make these changes without his help. Many times we look for relief from people, things, or substances. That is why God gave us spiritual armor.

Paul instructs, "Put on all of God's armor so that you will be able to stand firm against all strategies of the devil" (Ephesians 6:11). Satan will try to trick us. He will make us believe God's ways are not best for us by lying or distorting reality. Satan twisted the Lord's command when he spoke to Eve in the garden of Eden (Genesis 3:1), and he twisted God's words when he talked to Jesus in the desert (Matthew 4:5–6), so don't you think Satan will distort truth to trick us too?

Similarly, when we go to the grocery store, many foods that are harmful are labeled natural, healthy, low-fat, and whole-grain because the food industry wants us to think the food is nutritious. The twisting of the truth makes it seem legitimate.

Truth twisting also takes place in our minds, sometimes from a spiritual attack. Examples include negative self-talk, self-doubt, or not forgiving oneself for binging (even after you asked to be forgiven). This is like a demon sitting on your shoulder, whispering destructive thoughts.

Resist the lies of the enemy when he tells you that you will fail. You are a child of God and have the Holy Spirit inside of you, who is greater than Satan. Stand by the commitment you made to God in session 1 to improve your health and eat his foods. However, you are going to need God's armor to fend off an attack from the enemy.

DAY 4: THE ARMOR OF GOD

God equipped us with spiritual weapons so we could use his power to fight the enemy. We can resist our opponent and his army by using the biblical arsenal, the armor of God. The seven components of the armor include:

- Belt of truth—accepting God's moral standards as our own.
- Breastplate of righteousness—living our life by God's standards, his truth.
- Shoes of good news of peace—we receive God's peace when we believe, trust, and obey God's Word; this is the assurance of the gospel of Jesus Christ.
- Shield of faith—believing God is telling us the truth. Faith is our shield.
- Helmet of salvation—believing Jesus Christ is our Savior.
- Sword of the Spirit—knowing, applying, and speaking the Word of God.
- Prayer—asking God to intervene on our behalf.

The first five weapons are defensive arms, which protect us from an enemy's attack. The last two weapons are offensive and used to attack our opponent.

Belt of Truth and Breastplate of Righteousness

Our first defensive weapon, the belt of truth, is accepting God's moral standards as our own. We need the belt of truth to stand firm against temptation. When we choose the Lord's morals, we put on his belt, which will protect us from Satan—a roaring lion, looking for someone to devour (1 Peter 5:8).

The breastplate of righteousness, our second defensive weapon, is obtained through living our life by the Lord's standards. It is accepting his morals as our values. Living our life in obedience to those values is wearing the breastplate of righteousness.

We become righteous when we ask him to forgive us of our sins and accept Jesus Christ as our Lord and Savior; at that moment God replaces our sin with our Savior's righteousness—since he never sinned. To learn more about accepting Jesus, see Appendix 7: How to Become a Christian and Disciple of Jesus Christ in *7 Steps to Get Off Sugar and Carbohydrates*.

The belt of truth is God's ethical principles, and the breastplate of righteousness is living by those standards or at least attempting to. We all fail to hit the mark, yet we should try. When we fail, we repent (ask the Lord for forgiveness and turn away from sin), which places us back in right standing with him.

If we choose not to repent, then we become unrighteous, which gives Satan an invitation to mess with us. Sin removes God's protective breastplate. Satan's army will tempt us not to walk out the Lord's standards in our life. If Satan succeeds, this opens a door for him and demons to enter, influence, and control our lives. Instead, we need to submit to God's truth as our standard and live by it. Paul explains this in Romans 6:16: "Don't you realize that you become the slave of whatever you choose to obey? You can be a slave to sin, which leads to death, or you can choose to obey God, which leads to righteous living."

In your own words, please explain how the belt of truth and breastplate of righteousness are interconnected? Are you wearing these defensive weapons?

Shoes of Good News of Peace

The third defensive weapon, the shoes of the good news of peace, follows when our mind agrees with, and we live by, God's principles outlined in his Word. The Holy Spirit, whom we received at salvation, helps us want to obey God and gives us access to his power and peace. Even though our human nature influences us to do wrong, the Holy Spirit gives us the desire to obey God and convicts us when we don't.

If our mind agrees with the Lord's moral standards—his truth— and we obey, we receive the shoes of peace. These shoes make us stable so that during difficult circumstances we retain God's peace. Calmness and tranquility will exist in the midst of chaos and trouble. Even though Satan will try to knock us off our feet, if we wear the shoes of peace, we continue to stand.

When we experience fear and anxiety, and peace is not our typical way to function, then we may be out of sync spiritually. As we wear the belt of truth and live by it, we display calm confidence and trust in Jesus Christ with a spirit of peace.

Does your mind agree with and follow the principles provided for us in the Bible? Do you feel double-minded or lack peace in your life?

Shield of Faith

God gave us the shield of faith as our fourth defensive weapon in his artillery. The shield is our faith. Faith is what we believe; it is part of the unseen realm. We access the Lord's power if we have faith and believe that his power is within us through the Holy Spirit. Believe that "the one who is in you is greater than the one who is in the world" (1 John 4:4 NIV).

Satan targets the most vulnerable areas of our lives, such as our palate and cravings. When you feel the attack, pick up the shield of faith and stop those fiery arrows. Faithfulness believes we will overcome through God's strength within us.

Even though we may experience setbacks, we can win the healthy living war. Once you falter, get back to doing what you know is right. Faith is our shield, and it shows up in the way we live our lives.

When you ask God to help you when you are tempted, do you believe he will support you? Do you ask him for help as often as you should? Write a prayer below asking for his aid in the areas you need and for more faith.

. . .

Helmet of Salvation

Our fifth defensive weapon is the helmet of salvation. Salvation happens when we recognize our sinfulness and ask the Lord to forgive us. We accept that Jesus humbled himself in obedience to God by dying on a cross to pay for our sins. Since Jesus never sinned, he was an acceptable sacrifice to pay the debt (eternal damnation) for our sins. Once we accept Christ's gift and ask him to come into our hearts, we are filled with the Holy Spirit. Accepting Jesus places the helmet of salvation on our heads. Our Savior's Spirit within us gives us the ability to tap into God's supernatural power.

In your own words, write out the meaning of the helmet of salvation.

When we accept Christ as our Savior, God adopts us as his children and loves us unconditionally, like a devoted parent. Nothing can take his love away from us. Since we are his children, we can access his power by faith and apply it to any area in our lives.[4] Satan does not want us to believe we can tap into the Lord's power or have faith in Jesus. Instead, he tries to gain access to our minds, through deception and twisting of the truth (God's moral standards), because whatever controls our minds controls our lives.

Satan wants you to believe that just because you were gluttonous you are a failure. He will try to discourage you so you doubt your worth. The enemy wants you to focus on losing the last battle versus winning the war. Have faith that through God's strength you will succeed in overcoming your plight with food.

The devil wants to fill our thoughts with doubt, lies, and discouragement—like when we give up on eating well because we binged. We must fight Satan's tactics and the norms of this world, and be obedient to the Lord; only then can we effectively combat the demonic realm. If Satan controls our thoughts, he controls us, and he desires this greatly. Therefore, wrestle the enemy with God's strength, not your willpower.

DAY 5: OFFENSIVE SPIRITUAL WEAPONS

The last two weapons in the armor of God are offensive: the sword of the Spirit and prayer. The Greek word for this sword is *macaira*, a short sword, like a dagger. A Roman soldier used this type of weapon when his defensive armaments were unsuccessful. After his shield and other armor were lost, he pulled out his short blade for hand-to-hand combat with his enemy because a dagger could provide a death blow to a vital organ.[5]

Sword of the Spirit

Spoken Bible verses have the power to do whatever they state. Scripture is the sword of the Spirit, and Satan has been trying to dull this blade from the beginning (with Eve in the garden of Eden).[6] However, the devil can't stand against the dominant force of the spoken Word of God.

Jesus showed us how to use this offensive weapon. When he fasted for forty days in the desert, Satan knew he was physically weak and hungry, so he suggested Jesus turn stones into bread. Again the devil tempted with food. Jesus replied, "For the Scriptures say" followed by an Old Testament verse. Jesus stabbed Satan with God's Word three different times, and then Satan left. If our Savior needed to use scripture to defeat Satan, shouldn't we rely on this crucial weapon too?

The sword of the Spirit torments demons:

> When Jesus stepped ashore, he was met by a demon-possessed man from the town. For a long time this man had not worn clothes or lived in a house, but had lived in the tombs. When he saw Jesus, he cried out and fell at his feet, shouting at the top of his voice, "What do you want with me, Jesus, Son of the Most High God? I beg you, don't torture me!"

> Luke 8:27–28 (NIV)

We can torture evil spirits by speaking Bible verses out loud. Isn't that amazing! When Jesus did this, Satan left. The blade of the spoken Word of God slices into the invisible realm. It cuts demonic forces we cannot see. We must use God's arsenal and not rely solely on human resources to defeat our enemy.

Another component of using the sword of the Spirit is to be in sync with the Holy Spirit (who lives inside of us) when operating this offensive weapon. The sword will not be useful if we approach the spiritual battle from our emotions, desires, or vengeful tendencies. Instead, we need to be quiet and pray, or praise the Lord through music, until we feel connected to the Holy Spirit within us. When we are spiritually connected is the time to proclaim Bible verses out loud, and this spiritual dagger will stab the enemy. It is the Spirit who uses the sword through us. Tap into the spiritual realm, because part of our being is spirit.

To succeed in conquering your palate and overcoming temptation, it is essential to know, apply, and speak God's Word. Effective use of this weapon requires becoming familiar with Bible verses so we can employ them in battle. For example: when experiencing fear, speak,

"For God has not given us a spirit of fear and timidity, but of power, love, and self-discipline" (2 Timothy 1:7). Next time you ponder a negative thought, look up an opposing Bible verse to the idea and speak the scripture out loud.

Prayer

Prayer is our second offensive weapon. When we pray, we give earthly permission for God to intervene on our behalf. When life gets tough, and we experience pain and anguish, we should pray instead of turning to human products to relieve our tension. Our Lord gives us everything we need to cope with any stress that life or Satan fires at us. If we ask the Lord to help us, he will provide us with his power and strength to resist the enemy.

We should also use Jesus's name when we pray because Jesus told us, "I tell you the truth, you will ask the Father directly, and he will grant your request because you use my name. You haven't done this before. Ask, using my name, and you will receive, and you will have abundant joy" (John 16:23–24). When we use Jesus's name as we pray, we evoke his spiritual authority.

Do you use Jesus's name when asking God for something through prayer? If not, do you plan on doing this in the future?

Before we pray we should confess our sins, because as Psalm 66:18 reminds us, "If I had not confessed the sin in my heart, the Lord would not have listened." Therefore, if we don't come clean before God, he may not listen to our prayer. If a person overeats to the point of gluttony, he or she sins. Every time you overeat, bring this infraction to the Lord and ask him to forgive you and help you overcome temptation.

Do you have a confession to make to the Lord? If yes, write it below.

_____

_____

Satan would prefer for you to succumb to the temptation to overeat. Make a commitment right now that you will confess each time you sin through gluttony and get back on track, knowing that you are forgiven and empowered to finish the race.

Write your commitment below.

_____

_____

This commitment is similar to the consistency needed when disciplining a child. To be effective we must teach ourselves to repent every time. If we repent immediately, we stop the sin (yeast) before it has a chance to grow.

So next time you sin, ask Jesus to forgive you as soon as you realize it. If you are genuinely sorry and will try your best to turn away from that sin, he will forgive you. "God is faithful and reliable.

When we confess our sins, he forgives them and cleanses us from everything we've done wrong" (John 1:9 GW).

After we repent, God immediately takes away the sin, and we are clean again. In fact, he chooses not to remember our sins anymore, as Hebrews 8:12 states, "For I will be merciful regarding their wrong deeds, and I will never again remember their sins" (ISV). Isn't it wonderful to know the Lord does not keep a record of our offenses? Instead, he chooses not to remember them.

Using God's Armor

During the past two days, we learned how to employ seven spiritual weapons from the armor of God. The belt of truth is God's moral standards, and the breastplate of righteousness is living out those standards. The shield of faith believes what God tells us is accurate and in our best interest. We wear the shoes of good news of peace when we wear the belt and breastplate, because our minds are peaceful as we live out what we believe.

Our fifth defensive weapon, the helmet of salvation, occurs when we recognize our sinfulness and ask the Lord to forgive us. We accept that Jesus died in our place as a substitute for the consequences of our sins. Once we accept his gift of salvation and ask him to come into our hearts, we are filled with the Holy Spirit, which gives us the ability to tap into God's supreme power. Accepting Jesus as our Lord and Savior places the helmet of salvation on our heads.

We have two offensive weapons we can use to attack Satan: the sword of the Spirit and prayer. The sword of the Spirit is knowing, applying, and speaking the Word of God. Prayer is when we call on the Lord and ask for him to intervene on our behalf. Paul tells us to "put on all of God's armor."

Do you wear all seven pieces of the armor? Which piece do you need to work on and why?

. . .

_____

_____

To use the armor of God, first we must become his warrior through accepting Jesus as our Lord. When he becomes the leader of our life, we gain the extraordinary power to fight sin, which is like having a superpower. Then we can outlast the enemy by using the Lord's power within us.

Session 5 Action Steps

Accessing God's power is crucial for maintaining this new way of eating. Take these action steps listed below:

1. Implement the Seven-Day Eating Plan listed in appendix 6 of *7 Steps to Get Off Sugar and Carbohydrates*. Go to SusanUNeal.com/appendix for a printable version of the all the appendices. Date you will start this plan (remember to start on a Wednesday): _____.
2. Plan for the pitfalls. Print the list of Food Addiction Battle Strategies from appendix 10 of *7 Steps to Get Off Sugar and Carbohydrates*, and use these strategies as you stumble.
3. Implement the Five-Step Binding the Strong Man Plan and print a copy of the plan (appendix 8 of *7 Steps to Get Off Sugar and Carbohydrates*).
4. Choose a specific verse to use when the strong man of addiction tempts you. Write the verse on an index card and memorize it.
5. Continue to record pertinent information in your journal such as: what food problems have been with you since

childhood, and what are you grateful for (see the Gratitude Log in the *Healthy Living Journal*).

6. Every time you overeat, immediately confess your sin to God.

7. If you are not wearing the full armor of God, work on the areas where you are weak.

PART VI

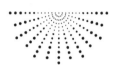

SESSION 6: PREPARE AND EAT FOOD DIFFERENTLY

Five weeks slipped by; you only have one more week before you complete the study. Last week was challenging as you implemented the Seven-Day Eating Plan and fought temptation through the Five-Step Binding the Strong Man Plan. Did you feel like you were in a battle? I did.

Did you implement the Seven-Day Eating Plan? If yes, share your experience with the group.

Have you started taking the anti-Candida cleanse? If yes, how is that going?

. . .

Share with the group how effective you found the Binding the Strong Man Plan for fighting temptation.

In today's session, you will learn tips to guide you, so you can continue this healthy eating journey for the rest of your life. But first, discuss the fill-in-the-blank questions from days 1–5 and the action steps listed at the end of session 5. (*Leader: discuss session 5 questions before proceeding.*)

Next read the sixth chapter of *7 Steps to Get Off Sugar and Carbohydrates*, Step 6: Prepare and Eat Foods Differently. Skip the Meal Planning and Menu Planning sections, as participants will read these on their own. Each member can read one paragraph or section out loud to the group. Whatever portion of the chapter you are not able to finish should be assigned as homework. Ask the following questions after reading each section.

Only Eat until You're Full

To be in tune with the sensation of fullness and decrease your portion size, what tactics will you implement?

Eating Out

What tips do you plan to apply so you can eat healthy items at a fast-food restaurant and not overeat at a full-service restaurant?

. . .

Follow the Healthy Eating Guidelines

Which healthy eating guideline do you find difficult to follow? Why?

Curb Your Sweet Tooth

Curbing your sweet tooth can be challenging, therefore, what suggestions do you plan to try?

Spiritual Preparation

From this section, what spiritual tactic did you find most helpful?

Conclusion

During the past five weeks, you gained knowledge and self-confidence as you learned to wield God's power through the Holy Spirit. Now you can apply the healthy living tips in this chapter to remain on course. You are changing your future for the better by taking the journey to improve your health. I am proud of you and God is too.

DAY 1: CREATE YOUR STANDARDIZED GROCERY LIST

Lack of planning can cause an individual to stumble. Therefore, it is vital to take the time to create a weekly menu with a corresponding grocery list. By doing this you avoid eating something unhealthy because you did not have fresh foods available.

Read the section titled Meal Planning and Menu Planning in chapter 6 of *7 Steps to Get Off Sugar and Carbohydrates*. Also from the *7 Steps* book, peruse Appendix 4: Recipes. Then create your menu for the week.

Be sure to include healthy snacks from the Curb the Sweet Tooth section in the sixth chapter. My favorite snack is almond butter slathered on green apple slices. Post your menu on the refrigerator, so you know what you need to do to prepare for each meal.

If you didn't create your standardized shopping list based on the grocery store you usually visit, please create it now (see session 4, day 1, Menu Planning). See the appendix in this study guide for an example of a list. Each week, print a new grocery list and add items to the list as you run out. This method will streamline your grocery store planning.

. . .

What obstacles do you face in creating a weekly menu and shopping list? How can you address theses challenges to start a new way of food planning?

_____

_____

Who in your family can you enlist to help you in menu planning and/or shopping? How can they partner with you to help?

_____

_____

DAY 2: IMPLEMENT ACTION STEPS FROM STEPS 1–2

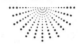

We covered a great deal of material in the past six weeks. To help you succeed in getting off sugar and carbohydrates, action steps were included at the end of each chapter in this Christian study guide and in *7 Steps to Get Off Sugar and Carbohydrates*. The next four days will focus on ensuring that you implemented all those action steps. Please put a check mark beside each action step after you finish it and plan a non-food-related treat (massage, facial, manicure, vacation, new swimsuit/outfit) for yourself after you completed *all* the steps in each section.

Taking Step 1: Decide (from *7 Steps to Get Off Sugar and Carbohydrates*)

Deciding to commit to a lifestyle change, particularly if you struggle with food addiction, is crucial. From step 1, review the following action steps and check them off once you've accomplished each one:

1. If you haven't already, watch the Ted-Ed video, "How Does

Sugar Affect the Brain?" by the neuroscientist Nicole Avena, Ph.D.: https://www.sciencealert.com/watch-this-is-how-sugar-affects-your-brain.

2. Check labels to make sure you don't consume sugary foods with greater than 10 grams of sugar per serving.
3. Write and sign your contract between you and God.
4. Complete your assessments.

Action Steps (from session 1 of this study guide)

1. Read the introduction and first chapter (Step 1: Decide to Improve Your Health) in *7 Steps to Get Off Sugar and Carbohydrates.*
2. Acquire a prayer/accountability partner and sign your commitment together.
3. Request to join the closed Facebook group: 7 Steps to Get Off Sugar and Carbohydrates.
4. Create a commitment between you and God.
5. Don't eat anything with greater than 10 grams of sugar at one sitting.
6. Stop eating refined carbohydrates such as snacks you find in boxes and bags.
7. Take a food addiction test.
8. Drag your skeleton out of the closet and share it with your small group.
9. Write your Bible verse on an index card or under the notes app in your cell phone.
10. Express to God the struggle you experience with food and surrender this issue to Jesus.

From completing the steps in step 1, on a scale of 1–10, rank the resolve or commitment to changing your lifestyle that you experienced.

Taking Step 2: Acquire (from *7 Steps to Get Off Sugar and Carbohydrates*)

You are well on your way to becoming a healthier person. Review your progress on the suggested action steps from this chapter:

1. Take the food addiction test.
2. If you have a food addiction, join a Christian weight loss or food addiction program.
3. Conduct the Candida spit test.
4. Take the gluten-sensitivity test by eliminating wheat for one month, and then reintroduce it into your diet to see if you experience any ill effects.
5. Choose an accountability/prayer partner if you haven't yet done so.
6. Join my closed Facebook group, 7 Steps to Get Off Sugar and Carbohydrates to gain additional support.
7. Purchase a journal and start recording the items listed in appendix 3.
8. Choose a scripture verse to fight temptation, write it on an index card, and memorize it.

Action Steps (from session 2 of this study guide)

1. Read the second chapter of *7 Steps to Get Off Sugar and*

Carbohydrates, Step 2: Acquire a Support System and Knowledge.

2. Plan your menu and grocery list for the week.
3. Only eat organic corn, wheat, oat, soy, and beet products because of the potential carcinogenic glyphosate residue.
4. Avoid eating wheat.
5. Record your food and activity for this week in your journal. The *Healthy Living Journal* has a Daily Food Journal chart for you to complete.
6. Conduct the Candida spit test. If it is positive, purchase an anti-Candida cleanse.

Since acquiring knowledge about harmful foods, what has been the most difficult food to give up? Have you found a replacement for that food item? What alternatives do you plan to try?

_____

_____

_____

DAY 3: IMPLEMENT ACTION STEPS
FROM STEPS 3–4

Did you complete most of the action steps from day 2? It takes time to finish everything, especially the gluten-sensitivity test where you need to eliminate wheat for a month. Do you enjoy checking items off the list? I do! Also, accomplishing these tasks boosts a person's self-worth.

How does it make you feel when you accomplish each task? Do you feel more confident that you can undertake the next task too?

_____

Listed below are the action steps for steps 3 and 4 from this Christian study guide and *7 Steps to Get Off Sugar and Carbohydrates*. Put a check mark beside each step after you complete it.

Taking Step 3: Clean Out (from *7 Steps to Get Off Sugar and Carbohydrates*)

Now that you've made it to step 3, you should feel more confident about incorporating new food choices into your healthy lifestyle. Make sure you took the following action steps:

1. Schedule a date to clean out your pantry, refrigerator, and freezer.

Date to clean out:

Pantry _____

Refrigerator _____

Freezer _____

2. Cleaning out your emotions entails several steps. Do you have a journal yet? Are you journaling what you eat and determining why you are eating when you are not hungry? Please see appendix 3 for the list of items you should be recording in your journal, or order the *Healthy Living Journal*. Be sure to journal your thoughts and emotions too.
3. Record the things in your life that cause you stress.
4. Think about ways you can reduce or eliminate these stressors.
5. List some activities you would like to do to decrease your stress.

Action Steps (from session 3 of this study guide)

1. Read the third chapter of *7 Steps to Get Off Sugar and Carbohydrates*, Step 3: Clean Out the Pantry and Refrigerator.

2. Clean out your pantry, refrigerator, and freezer.
3. Clean out your emotions with God by telling him what you think is the origin of your unhealthy eating habits and ask him to help you heal from any emotional scars.
4. Fully commit your heart to the Lord.
5. Determine the stressors (things that cause you stress) in your life, and figure out how to minimize them.
6. If you need to forgive someone, do one of the activities suggested in day 5 of session 3.
7. Share your forgiveness story with your small group.

Since implementing the steps above, have you successfully decreased stress in your life? What additional actions can you take to eliminate stressors?

_____

_____

Did you undertake one of the forgiveness activities in day 5 of session 3? If yes, did you experience a new level of forgiveness? What was that like for you?

_____

_____

. . .

Taking Step 4: Purchase (from *7 Steps to Get Off Sugar and Carbohydrates*)

Step 4 helps you plan and purchase healthy foods so you eat God's provisions. Make sure you completed the following action steps:

1. Become familiar with the healthy eating guidelines provided in step 4 and appendix 5. Print out a printable version of this appendices at SusanUNeal.com/appendix.
2. Determine what alternatives you will use for sugar, pasta, dairy, and to some extent, meat.
3. Plan your menu for the week and a corresponding grocery list. Join my blog at SusanUNeal.com/healthy-living-blog to find menus and grocery lists.
4. Purchase healthy organic fruits, vegetables, whole grains, nuts, seeds, fish, and meats.
5. If needed, buy an anti-Candida cleanse.
6. If you haven't done so already, purchase a journal and record the items from appendix 3.

Action Steps (from session 4 of this study guide)

1. Read the fourth chapter of *7 Steps to Get Off Sugar and Carbohydrates*, Step 4: Purchase Healthy Foods and an Anti-Candida Cleanse.
2. Prepare your menu and corresponding grocery list.
3. Purchase healthy foods.
4. If needed, buy an anti-Candida cleanse.
5. Take a probiotic supplement.
6. Do not purchase or eat processed foods out of boxes and bags.
7. Replace some servings of meat with alternative protein sources.

8. Train yourself to bring every negative thought to Jesus and ask him to remove it from your mind.
9. On bad days, focus on your victories not your failures.
10. Record new healthy living habits in your journal.

Have you eaten less processed foods since implementing these steps? If yes, what have you eaten instead?

_____

What type of alternative protein sources have you tried? What else do you plan to try?

_____

How successful have you been in bringing every negative thought to Jesus and asking him to remove it? Renewing the mind is an essential part of changing your lifestyle. How can you remind yourself to do this more often?

_____

_____

_____

DAY 4: IMPLEMENT ACTION STEPS FROM STEPS 5–6

As you near the finish line, Paul's words may encourage you, "So let's not get tired of doing what is good. At just the right time we will reap a harvest of blessing if we don't give up" (Galatians 6:9). You can get off sugar and carbohydrates and implement the steps in this book!

Don't give up. Instead, reestablish the commitment you made to God, so you can accomplish the work he has for you. We are the hands and feet of Christ to accomplish his purpose on Earth. You may stumble—we all do—but with the help of Christ you can make these much-needed lifestyle changes. I am praying you will.

Do you stumble over the same issue over and over again? If yes, what is the obstacle? Pray and ask God to help you formulate a solution to the problem and write his answer below.

. . .

Remember to use the sword of the Spirit when tempted. Call your prayer partner as needed, and confess your flub-ups to this person and the Lord. Accountability helps keep a person on the right track. Stay connected with your small group by attending the weekly study for this book. That sense of connection and understanding that you are not the only person who struggles will help you "not get tired of doing what is good."

How do you feel about changes that are happening, if not physically, then maybe mentally or emotionally or spiritually during our five weeks together?

Taking Step 5: Implement the Physical and Spiritual Plans (from *7 Steps to Get Off Sugar and Carbohydrates*)

Planning is crucial for maintaining this new lifestyle. Review your progress on these action steps:

1. Implement the Seven-Day Eating Plan listed in appendix 6. Print out appendix 6.
2. Plan for the pitfalls. Print the list of Food Addiction Battle Strategies from appendix 10, and use these strategies as you stumble.
3. Implement the Five-Step Binding the Strong Man Plan and print a copy of the plan (appendix 8).
4. Choose a specific verse to use when the strong man of addiction tempts you. Write the verse on an index card and memorize it.
5. Continue to record pertinent information in your journal (such as: what food problems have you experienced since childhood), and list all you can praise and thank God for and express your gratitude to him.

Action Steps (from session 5 of this study guide)

1. Steps 1–4 are the same as listed above.
2. Every time you overeat, immediately confess your sin to the Lord.
3. If you are not wearing the full armor of God, work on the areas where you are weak.

How successful have you been with confessing your sin of overeating? Once you ask for forgiveness, he chooses not to remember your sins. How can you remind yourself to repent more often? (You should journal each episode in the Binge Eating Tracker in the *Healthy Living Journal*.)

· · ·

Taking Step 6: Prepare (from *7 Steps to Get Off Sugar and Carbohydrates*)

This step helps you prepare for a new way of eating and provides a spiritual strategy for the changes you are making. Finish the action steps listed below:

1. Plan your menu for the week and post it on the refrigerator.
2. Create a standardized grocery list that you can print out every week when planning your menu.
3. Go grocery shopping.
4. Prepare healthy meals from scratch using the Healthy Eating Guidelines in appendix 5.
5. Pay attention to: portion control and water intake
6. Eat fresh and raw items at fast-food restaurants.
7. Use techniques to curb your sweet tooth (see appendix 9).
8. Continue to record pertinent information in your journal. Through using this journal have you identified your food triggers? Do you have a plan for how to reduce those triggers? Have you told yourself lies that justify inappropriate eating? Journal those lies. Replace those lies with the Word of God.
9. Memorize one scripture verse per week. Choose the verse, write it on an index card, and memorize it.
10. Download and use the app "I Deserve a Donut and Other Lies That Make You Eat" by Barb Raveling.

Have you ordered healthy menu items at restaurants yet? When served a large entrée, did you try the portion control method of deciding how much to take home before you started eating?

_____

_____

Has drinking more water decreased your appetite? Do you drink the recommended amount of water for your weight? If not, how do you plan to increase your consumption of water?

_____

_____

_____

DAY 5: IMPLEMENT ACTION STEPS FROM STEP 7

Congratulations on taking all these steps to improve your health, life, and future! As you continue with these lifestyle changes, utilize the following actions steps:

Taking Step 7: Improve your Health (from *7 Steps to Get Off Sugar and Carbohydrates*)

1. Remember the 80/20 percent rule. If you improve your eating 80 percent of the time, you will improve your diet and health. However, healing takes time, so be patient.
2. Expect to stumble. No one is perfect; give yourself grace, as God does, when you mess up and eat poorly.
3. Rely on God. Turn to him and the Bible verses you memorized when you stumble.
4. Document your path to recovery in your journal. How do you look at food? Are you using food to comfort and meet an emotional need, or do you think of food as a necessity to keep your body functioning? Have you journaled about

this? Do you turn to food to help you deal with the challenges of life? If so, food is your stronghold. Learn from your mistakes as you record what occurred, and figure out why so you can prevent these mishaps in the future.

5. Hand over control of your eating habits to the Lord. Relinquish the outcome of your lifestyle change to God. Submit your life to him. Live in victory through total reliance on him.

6. Mark a date on your calendar to perform a self-assessment six months into your journey. Compare this assessment to the first one you took at the beginning of this journey. Note your areas of improvement in the Victory Log in the *Healthy Living Journal* and let these victories motivate you to continue to improve and maintain your new healthy lifestyle.

In what ways have you found your journal helpful?

Relinquishing control or your lifestyle change to God is another key component to success. Have you done this yet? If not write a prayer below and hand control over to him.

.   .   .

Recently I ate a chia/oatmeal breakfast bowl with berries while my daughter ate eggs benedict over biscuits. Her meal looked more appetizing than my mush bowl. I could have eaten the eggs benedict on spinach, but I had already prepared my dish. Eating healthy reminded me of the hard work a person does to groom themselves. A man shaves his face and plucks his nose hairs. A woman shaves her legs, plucks her eyebrows, and applies makeup. Looking attractive takes a great deal of work. Have you ever heard the saying "No pain, no gain"?

Eating well takes effort too, but the rewards are marvelous when you can fit back into a slenderizing outfit, or feel like a healthier you. One woman commented, "I looked great after I lost all that weight and my husband was actually attentive." When you look good physically, it changes the way you and others feel about you.

After making this lifestyle change, you will feel better emotionally, not just about what you see in the mirror. Looking and feeling healthier will change the way you think of yourself, even if you haven't lost as much weight as you would like. Your self-esteem will rise.

Once you gain control of dysfunctional eating habits, your relationship with God will improve too. You will obtain an intrinsic sense of value from being a good steward of the body he gave you. Family members will be proud of your efforts too. Your renewed energy level and stamina will allow you to keep up with family members during fun activities. Family relationships will improve. In fact, your physical, emotional, and spiritual well-being will soar. Continue to eat God's foods, and you will reap all the benefits he desires for you.

PART VII

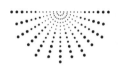

PART VII

SESSION 7: IMPROVE YOUR HEALTH

Congratulations on completing the study. I am proud of you! Is your body thanking you for treating it as a temple and feeding it the food from the Lord's bounty? Are you feeling better? In this session you will compare the symptoms checklist you filled out in session 1 with how you feel today, but first let's discuss the action steps from days 1–5 in session 6. (*Leader: discuss session 6 questions before proceeding, but ask participants to list the steps they have not completed in the space provided below.*)

What steps do you have left to complete from each area? Note the date you plan to do each unfinished task.

Step 1: _____

Step 2: _____

. . .

Step 3: _____

Step 4: _____

Step 5: _____

Step 6: _____

Step 7: _____

Next read the seventh chapter of *7 Steps to Get Off Sugar and Carbohydrates*, Step 7: Improve Your Health. Each member can read one paragraph or section out loud to the group. Whatever portion of the chapter you are not able to finish should be assigned as homework. Ask the following questions after reading each section.

Give Yourself Grace

What do you think of the 80/20 percent rule? Has it helped you?

_____

Have you experienced an all-or-nothing attitude about eating when you messed up, so you continued to eat poorly for the rest of the day?

_____

. . .

When you give yourself grace after you eat something you know you should not eat, are you able to turn the day around and eat healthy for the rest of the day? Why or why not?

_____

_____

Let Your Mistakes Motivate You

Have you identified a food that causes you to feel foggy brained and experience low energy? If yes, share with the group the food that caused these undesirable symptoms.

_____

Food Addiction Revisited

What food triggers have you identified that you need to avoid? How are you avoiding them?

_____

_____

Benefits of Healthy Eating

What was the first negative symptom to go away once you began eating natural, organic foods? Have additional symptoms been resolved or improved? Explain.

. . .

_____

_____

The Path to Recovery and Health

Have you identified the root cause of a dysfunctional eating behavior? How has this study helped to heal that issue? If it hasn't, what next step can you take in this area?

_____

_____

Did you use any of the Food Addiction Battle Strategies listed in appendix 10 of the *7 Steps* book ? If yes, which one, and how was it helpful? (You can obtain a printable version of the appendices at SusanUNeal.com/appendix.)

_____

_____

Turn to God

Have you relinquished control of your lifestyle change to the Lord and relied on his power to evoke change? If not, what is stopping you?

If yes, how hard was it to give up control? What difference has it made in keeping your commitment to a healthier lifestyle?

Seven-Week Self-Assessment

Date:

Weight:

Waistline:

Symptom Checklist
Put a check by the unhealthy symptoms you still experience.

_____ Fatigue
_____ Anxiety
_____ Insomnia
_____ Irritability
_____ Depression
_____ Mood swings
_____ Poor memory

_____ Food allergies

_____ Foggy brained

_____ Decreased sex drive

_____ Hormonal imbalance

_____ Chronic fatigue, fibromyalgia

_____ Vaginal yeast infections, urinary tract infections

_____ Craving sweets and refined carbohydrates or alcohol

_____ Digestive issues (bloating, constipation, diarrhea) or disorders

_____ Skin and nail infections such as toenail fungus, athlete's foot, and ringworm

Compare this list to the same symptoms checklist in session 1. How many symptoms have been alleviated? Share with the group which symptoms improved.

_____

_____

Health Problems

Many health problems can keep you from an abundant life. Place a check mark by the following issues that improved in the past six weeks:

_____ Overweight

_____ Lack of energy

_____ Joint pain

_____ Ulcer

_____ Diabetes

_____ Allergies

_____ Sinus issues

_____ Take medication

_____ High blood pressure

_____ Autoimmune disease

_____ Bloating, gas, indigestion

_____ Constipation, diarrhea, or other gastrointestinal (GI) problem

_____ Skin problem—eczema, rosacea, rash

_____ Other _____

Share with the group which symptoms decreased.

_____

_____

Continue the Journey

You made significant progress, and you will continue to do so as you eat God's nutritious foods. Remember to evaluate everything you eat. If the food was not in the garden of Eden, don't eat it. Processed foods have no nutritional value, so consider them dead food. Instead, eat fresh raw vegetables, fruits, nuts, seeds, unrefined grains, and healthy sources of protein. Those are the foods our Creator originally designed for us.

Just think of how many more improvements your body will experience as it heals through eating the foods loaded in vitamins and minerals. The results of your six-month self-assessment should be astounding. Keep up the good work for the rest of your life, and receive all the blessings the Lord has in store for you.

If you need more guidance, I created the course, 7 Steps to Reclaim Your Health and Optimal Weight (SusanUNeal.com/courses/7-steps-to-get-off-sugar-and-carbs-course). This course will help you figure out and resolve the root cause of your inappropriate eating habits. One solved, taming your appetite is much easier. I show you how you can change your eating habits once and for all.

Ongoing Action Steps

1. Stay in contact with your prayer partner.
2. Keep writing in your *Healthy Living Journal.*
3. Touch base monthly with your study leader.
4. Learn and memorize a new scripture each month to help you continue to fight temptation.
5. Celebrate victories—reward yourself with something you enjoy that is not fattening! Like a spa day or a movie with a friend or prayer partner.
6. Continue to write your prayers to God.
7. Look for new recipes for healthy foods.
8. Perform another self-assessment in six months.

My greatest desire is that your health, weight, relationships, and life have improved. May God bless you and your endeavor to improve your health and well-being. Now go forth and serve the Lord!

Dear Heavenly Father,

Please bless each individual and group that completed this study. Help each one to achieve the results you want them to attain. Give them your supreme power so they can overcome the challenges they face. Hold them close to you, Lord, and fortify them with your redemptive strength. Jesus, through your holy name I pray. Amen.

APPENDIX

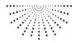

SAMPLE GROCERY LIST

This grocery list is based on my local store and is intended as a sample for you to create one based on the store or stores you shop at locally. Unhealthy foods may be listed here because many of us shop for other family members too.

Aisle 1 (Deli and Produce)
    Fruit juices, dried fruits, nuts
    Hummus, salsa, guacamole
    Produce

Aisle 2
    Granola bars, cereal, oatmeal
    Honey, syrup
    Coffee, tea

Aisle 3
    Mexican foods: salsa, tortillas

Hispanic and Asian food
Applesauce, canned fruits and soups
Tuna fish
Chocolate

Aisle 4

Bulk foods, trail mix, nuts
Sugar substitutes, sugar, baking chocolate
Baking goods, baking pans
Flour: coconut, almond, and gluten-free flours
Seasonings
Gluten-free pasta
Red Mill products
Pickles, Barbecue sauce, condiments, salad dressing, vinegar, oils

Aisle 5

Kitchen pots and pans
Canned vegetables
Spaghetti sauces
Dried beans, rice, pasta

Aisle 6

Iced tea, bottled water, coconut water, flavored waters, Gatorade,
soft drinks
Healthy granola bars
Greenwise (Publix's organic brand): honey; oatmeal; hemp, chia,
and flax seeds
Crackers, Goldfish, cookies, popcorn

Aisle 7

Potato chips

Bagged popcorn

Aisle 8
Office supplies, tape, glue, command hooks
Extension cords, batteries, flashlights
Cat and food, bowls, brushes, and supplies
Light bulbs, batteries
Dishwasher soap, sponges, gloves
Baking soda
Cleaning supplies

Aisle 9
Laundry detergent, bleach
Hangers, clothes pens, mothballs
Broom, mop, and cleaning devices
Bug sprays

Aisle 10
Frozen foods: dinners, potatoes, vegetables

Aisle 11
Frozen fruit bars, ice cream
Frozen fruit, frozen smoothie mixes
Frozen pizza
Wine

Aisle 12
Beer

. . .

Aisle 13
 Ziploc bags, aluminum foil, parchment paper, plastic wrap
 Trash bags, paper towel, napkins, paper plates/cups/utensils
 Kleenex, toilet paper

Aisle 14
 Baby supplies

Aisle 15
 Oral care, health and beauty supplies, soap

Aisle 16
 Dairy products
 Bread
 Nut butter
 Dried fruit

LEADER'S GUIDE

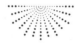

Ask participants to purchase *7 Steps to Get off Sugar and Carbohydrates* and the *Christian Study Guide for 7 Steps to Get off Sugar and Carbohydrates.* They also may want to purchase the corresponding *Healthy Living Journal.* These products can be purchased on Amazon.com or SusanUNeal.com/Shop.

Leader instructions are provided in *italics* throughout the book. The following suggestions may provide further guidance:

- Provide name tags for members.
- Start each session with prayer.
- Provide some sort of healthy snack at the beginning of each class. Recipes are included in appendix 4 of *7 Steps to Get Off Sugar and Carbohydrates.* You could ask members to rotate bringing a food item.
- During session 2, you could offer index cards for participants to write their strategic Bible verse on.
- While reading a chapter in *7 Steps to Get Off Sugar and*

Carbohydrates, look at the corresponding questions provided in that week's Christian study guide session. You may need to stop after reading one section in the *7 Steps* book and answer the question for that section from the study guide before moving on.

- Suggest that group members join the closed Facebook group: 7 Steps to Get Off Sugar and Carbohydrates.

May God bless your efforts to lead others to improve their health. If you have further questions, you may email me at SusanNeal@Bellsouth.net.

NOTES

Session 1

1. "Chronic Diseases: The Leading Causes of Death and Disability in the United States," Centers for Disease Control and Prevention, June 28, 2017, https://www.cdc.gov/chronicdisease/overview/index.htm.
2. Grace Donnelly, "Here's Why Life Expectancy in the U.S. Dropped Again This Year," *Fortune*, February 9, 2018, http://fortune.com/2018/02/09/us-life-expectancy-dropped-again/.
3. Fiona MacDonald, "Watch: This is How Sugar Affects Your Brain," *Science Alert*, November 3, 2015, Sciencealert.com/watch-this-is-how-sugar-affects-your-brain.
4. Fran Smith, "The Addicted Brain," *National Geographic*, September 2017, 36–37, 42–43.
5. Dale E. Bredesen, Edwin C. Amos, Jonathan Canick, Mary Ackerley, Cyrus Raji, Milan Fiala, and Jamila Ahdidan, "Reversal of cognitive decline in Alzheimer's disease," *Aging*, June 2016, http://www.aging-us.com/article/100981.

6. Ibid.

7. Deane Alban, "How to Increase Dopamine Naturally," Be Brain Fit, https://bebrainfit.com/increase-dopamine/.

8. Smith, "Addicted Brain," 36–37, 42–43.

Session 2

1. Alexander Lowen MD, *Narcissism: Denial of the True Self* (New York: Touchstone, 1997), 25, 79.

2. Timothy Keller, *The Freedom of Self-Forgetfulness* (Leyland, England: CPI Group, 2012), 16–17, 21–22.

3. Keller, *The Freedom of Self-Forgetfulness*, 31–32.

Session 3

1. "What's in Your Pantry?" by Tana Amen BSN, RN, and Dr. Daniel Amen, YouTube, https://www.youtube.com/watch?v=VqoWO0-RSAI.

2. Ibid.

3. Smith, "Addicted Brain," 51.

Session 4

1. "Candida Yeast Infection, Leaky Gut, Irritable Bowel and Food Allergies," National Candida Center, https://www.nationalcandidacenter.com/Leaky-Gut-and-Candida-Yeast-Infection-s/1823.htm.

2. Hannah Nichols, "The Top 10 Leading Causes of Death in

the United States," Medical News Today, February 23, 2017, https://www.medicalnewstoday.com/articles/282929.php.

3. Phillip Tusco MD, Scott R. Stoll MD, and William W. Li MD, "A Plant-Based Diet, Atherogenesis, and Coronary Artery Disease Prevention," *The Permanente Journal*, Winter 2015, https://www.ncbi.nlm.nih.gov/pmc/articles/PMC4315380/.

4. Joyce Meyer, *Battlefield of the Mind* (New York: Time Warner Book Group, 1995), 19–20, 28.

5. Ibid, 34.

Session 5

1. Smith, "Addicted Brain," 51.

2. Larry Lea, *The Weapons of Your Warfare: Equipping Yourself to Defeat the Enemy* (Reading, United Kingdom: Cox and Wyman, Ltd. 1990), 126, 182.

3. Joy A. Schneider, *Identifying the Hierarchy of Satan* (Fort Collins, Colorado: Water of Life Unlimited, 2002), 43.

4. Tony Evans, *Victory in Spiritual Warfare: Field Guide for Battle* (Nashville: B&H Publishing Group, 2011), 145.

5. Ibid, 153.

6. Ibid, 164–65.

HEALTHY LIVING JOURNAL

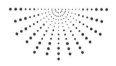

TRACK YOUR HEALTHY EATING AND LIVING
HABITS FOR IMPROVED HEALTH AND WELL-
BEING

Editor: Janis Whipple

Cover Design: Angie Alaya

Printed in the United States of America

ISBN: 978-0-997-76369-0

DISCLAIMER

Medical Disclaimer: This book offers health and nutritional information, which is for educational purposes only. The information provided in this book is designed to help individuals make informed decisions about their health; it is intended to supplement, not replace, the professional medical advice, diagnosis, or treatment of health conditions from a trained medical professional. Please consult your physician or healthcare provider before beginning or changing any health or eating habits to make sure that it is appropriate for you. If you have any concerns or questions about your health, you should always ask a physician or other healthcare provider. Please do not disregard, avoid, or delay obtaining medical or health-related advice from your healthcare professional because of something you may have read in this book. The author and publisher assume no responsibility for any injury that may result from changing your health or eating habits.

Disclaimer and Terms of Use: Every effort has been made to ensure the information in this book is accurate and complete. However, the author and publisher do not warrant the accuracy or completeness of the material, text, and graphics contained in this book. The author and publisher do not hold any responsibility for

errors, omissions, or contrary interpretation of the subject matter contained herein. This book is presented for motivational, educational, and informational purposes only. This book is sold with the understanding that the author and publisher are not engaged in rendering medical, legal, or other professional advice or services. Neither the publisher nor the author shall be liable for damages arising herein.

This book is dedicated to:

Edie Melson, for inspiring me to make this a journal with charts,
and
my daughter Shelby, for her encouragement, feedback, and help with
designing the charts.

JOURNAL BELONGS TO

This is the day that the LORD has made;
let us rejoice and be glad in it.
Psalm 118:24 (ESV)

This journal belongs to

_____

JOURNAL BENEFITS

Have you tried to decrease your weight or improve your health without success? Or maybe you lost the weight, but it came right back. This journal will help you make lifelong changes so you can reclaim the abundant life Jesus wants you to experience, not a life filled with disease and poor health.

This journal may help you:

- feel and look better
- increase energy
- grow in faith and grace
- sharpen clarity of mind
- harness God's strength to make changes
- become aware of negative food habits
- identify and eliminate behaviors that sabotage your health
- lose weight naturally without a fad diet or buying prepared meals and supplements

I hope you take this journey to improve your well-being.

2

HOW TO USE THIS JOURNAL

The *Healthy Living Journal* can be used independently or along with *7 Steps to Get Off Sugar and Carbohydrates*. Each day's entry helps you record daily water intake, exercise, and corresponding moods and energy. Recording your daily food consumption provides an opportunity to learn how food affects your health. When you discover negative health patterns you can change.

The first few logs and charts in this journal (located in the front of the book) will be used intermittently to track:

- Gratitude Log—things you are grateful for
- Victory Log—when you succeed in overcoming a food temptation, issue, or other pertinent item
- Blank Log—whatever you want
- Temptation/Struggle Log—things that tempt you to overeat and struggle with food
- Binge Eating Tracker—each time you binge and its corresponding effects
- Issue Tracker—undesirable health symptoms

- New Healthy Living Habits Log—each positive habit you want to incorporate into your life
- Blank Tracker—whatever you want

The Blank Log and Tracker are left blank for you to track you own specific issues.

The next three charts should be completed on a daily basis:

- Water Tracker
- Steps Tracker
- Fitness Tracker

The journal is divided into six weeks. Each week contains two charts that should be completed on a daily basis:

- Well-Being Chart
- Daily Food Journal

Color the corresponding boxes in the Well-Being Chart red when you experience negative symptoms and green when you experience positive symptoms. This will help you figure out what type of food makes your body function well or poorly.

Devotions and educational snippets are provided daily. Learn about food addiction, Candida infection of the gut, and healthy eating guidelines from these daily entries. As you gain knowledge, you will learn how to improve your health and weight. You will also journal and spend time with God. You are a child of God and deserve the most life has to offer you. Choose to take the time needed to improve your health; your body will thank you.

If you would like to dive deeper, a corresponding course, 7 Steps to Reclaim Your Health and Optimal Weight is available at Susan-UNeal.com/courses/7-steps-to-get-off-sugar-and-carbs-course. This course shows you how to use this book and *7 steps to Get Off Sugar and Carbohydrates* to meet your healthy living goals.

HEALTHY LIVING GOALS

Document the specific goals you would like to achieve.

Health

1.

2.

3.

Eating Habits

1.

2.

3.

Meal Planning

1.

2.

3.

Physical Activity

1.

2.

3.

Stress Relief

1.

2.

3.

Weight

1.

2.

3.

Sleep

1.

2.

3.

GOALS
ONE DAY AT A TIME
ONE MEAL AT A TIME
ONE WORKOUT AT A TIME

There is a time for everything,
and a season for every activity under the heavens.
Ecclesiastes 3:1 (NIV)

4

MEASUREMENTS

Document the specific goals you would like to achieve in reference to your measurements. However, seek progress not perfection.

1.

2.

3.

4.

5.

Measurements	Start Date	End Date
Upper Arms		
Chest		
Waist		
Hips		
Thighs		
Calves		
Weight		

SEEK PROGRESS
NOT PERFECTION

GRATITUDE LOG

Record things you are grateful for.

1.

2.

3.

4.

5.

6.

. . .

7.

8.

9.

10.

11.

12.

13.

14.

15.

Sing psalms and hymns and spiritual songs to God with thankful
hearts.
Colossians 3:16

6
VICTORY LOG

Record any victory you achieved, no matter how small it may be.

1.

2.

3.

4.

5.

6.

. . .

7.

8.

9.

10.

11.

12.

13.

14.

15.

The Lord is my strength and my song; he has given me **victory**. This
is my God, and I will praise him!
Exodus 15:2

7
BLANK LOG

TEMPTATION/STRUGGLE LOG

Determine if there is a pattern to your struggles by documenting the temptation here.

1.

2.

3.

4.

5.

6.

. . .

7.

8.

9.

10.

11.

12.

13.

14.

15.

And don't let us yield to **temptation**, but rescue us from the evil one.
Matthew 6:13

BINGE EATING TRACKER

Every time you binge, record the incident in the following Binge Eating Tracker chart. The items on the right side of the of the chart are for tracking your symptoms after you overate. Add a Y for yes and N for no for those items. Recognize if there is a correlation between energy level, mental clarity, and mood after binging. Also, note whether you experienced any digestive discomfort.

Determine your feelings before you binged and what temptation led you down that path. Did something trigger the episode? Figure out your trigger and record it in the Temptation/Struggle Log. After a while you may find a pattern—the same sort of situation or item tempts you. When you understand what entices you, you can learn to avoid it.

After binging, ask God to forgive you and help you not to binge again. Record your experience in the blank pages of the sixth or seventh day of each week's journal. These page are left blank to allow space for you to journal your thoughts and concerns.

If you record every incident of overeating in the following Binge Eating Tracker you will reduce the number of times you binge. Retraining your mind is like disciplining a child; consistency is vital to transformation. Ask God to help you along the way and he will.

Day	Time	Food	Qty.	Trigger /Why	Digestive Issue?	Low Energy Level?	Poor Mental Clarity?	Bad Mood?

Let us strip off every weight that slows us down, especially the sin that so easily trips us up. And let us run with endurance the race God has set before us.

Hebrews 12:1

ISSUE TRACKER

Whether you have a digestive issue or difficulty sleeping (it doesn't matter what the problem is), use this page to track when the issue occurs and what you ate up to twelve hours prior to the problem, so you can identify the culprit (example: foods containing MSG may disturb sleep or cause allergies).

DATE / PROBLEM / FOOD CONSUMED WITHIN 12 HRS

1.

2.

3.

4.

. . .

5.

6.

7.

8.

9.

10.

11.

12.

13.

14.

15.

Dear friend, I hope all is well with you and that you are as healthy in
body as you are strong in spirit.
3 John 2

NEW HEALTHY LIVING HABITS LOG

What new habits would you like to embrace?

1.

2.

3.

4.

5.

6.

. . .

7.

8.

9.

10.

11.

12.

13.

14.

15.

In everything you do, put God first, and he will direct you and crown
your efforts with success.
Proverbs 3:6 (TLB)

12

BLANK TRACKER

WATER TRACKER

It is essential to stay hydrated. However, we shouldn't appease our thirst with sugar-sweetened beverages because they fog the mind. Instead, we should drink the fluid God gave us—water. Our bodies desperately need water to flush out toxins and prevent dehydration.

The human body is comprised of 75 percent water, and we can't survive for more than a few days without it. Some people think drinking tea, juice, soda, or other drinks will hydrate their body, but they won't. In fact, caffeinated beverages are a diuretic, which cause you to urinate more frequently and lose fluids.

Water requirements depend upon your size. Various sources recommend: "Drink half your weight in ounces every day." Using this formula, a 130-pound person should drink eight glasses of water per day. (130/2 = 65 ounces; 65/8 ounces (1 cup) = 8 glasses.) Drink water in between meals, on an empty stomach, and up to fifteen minutes before you eat.

Day	Intake
1	◊◊◊◊◊◊◊◊◊
2	◊◊◊◊◊◊◊◊◊
3	◊◊◊◊◊◊◊◊◊
4	◊◊◊◊◊◊◊◊◊
5	◊◊◊◊◊◊◊◊◊
6	◊◊◊◊◊◊◊◊◊
7	◊◊◊◊◊◊◊◊◊
8	◊◊◊◊◊◊◊◊◊
9	◊◊◊◊◊◊◊◊◊
10	◊◊◊◊◊◊◊◊◊
11	◊◊◊◊◊◊◊◊◊
12	◊◊◊◊◊◊◊◊◊
13	◊◊◊◊◊◊◊◊◊
14	◊◊◊◊◊◊◊◊◊
15	◊◊◊◊◊◊◊◊◊
16	◊◊◊◊◊◊◊◊◊
17	◊◊◊◊◊◊◊◊◊
18	◊◊◊◊◊◊◊◊◊
19	◊◊◊◊◊◊◊◊◊
20	◊◊◊◊◊◊◊◊◊
21	◊◊◊◊◊◊◊◊◊

"For the Scriptures declare that rivers of living water shall flow from
the inmost being of anyone who believes in me."
John 7:38 (TLB)

Day	Intake
22	◊◊◊◊◊◊◊◊
23	◊◊◊◊◊◊◊◊
24	◊◊◊◊◊◊◊◊
25	◊◊◊◊◊◊◊◊
26	◊◊◊◊◊◊◊◊
27	◊◊◊◊◊◊◊◊
28	◊◊◊◊◊◊◊◊
29	◊◊◊◊◊◊◊◊
30	◊◊◊◊◊◊◊◊
31	◊◊◊◊◊◊◊◊
32	◊◊◊◊◊◊◊◊
33	◊◊◊◊◊◊◊◊
34	◊◊◊◊◊◊◊◊
35	◊◊◊◊◊◊◊◊
36	◊◊◊◊◊◊◊◊
37	◊◊◊◊◊◊◊◊
38	◊◊◊◊◊◊◊◊
39	◊◊◊◊◊◊◊◊
40	◊◊◊◊◊◊◊◊
41	◊◊◊◊◊◊◊◊
42	◊◊◊◊◊◊◊◊

14

STEPS TRACKER

Fitbits, Apple watches, and smartphones provide the wearer with the number of steps that they take each day. Technology is amazing, isn't it? But wearing all those devices can't make us get up and move. However, when you eat well, you feel better and this increase in energy can get you moving!

Every day record the number of steps you take either by coloring the boxes to notate the level of your steps or write the number of steps in the corresponding box.

After a week a two of eating well, you will get a new sense of energy. So get out there and walk, even if it is only down the block and back.

	Day 1	Day 2	Day 3	Day 4	Day 5	Day 6	Day 7	Day 8	Day 9	Day 10
10k										
9k										
8k										
8k										
7k										
6k										
5k										
4k										
3k										
2k										
1k										

The steps of good men are directed by the Lord. He delights in each step they take.

Psalm 37:23 (TLB)

	Day 11	Day 12	Day 13	Day 14	Day 15	Day 16	Day 17	Day 18	Day 19	Day 20	Day 21
10k											
9k											
8k											
8k											
7k											
6k											
5k											
4k											
3k											
2k											
1k											

	Day 22	Day 23	Day 24	Day 25	Day 26	Day 27	Day 28	Day 29	Day 30	Day 31
10k										
9k										
8k										
8k										
7k										
6k										
5k										
4k										
3k										
2k										
1k										

	Day 32	Day 33	Day 34	Day 35	Day 36	Day 37	Day 38	Day 39	Day 40	Day 41	Day 42
10k											
9k											
8k											
8k											
7k											
6k											
5k											
4k											
3k											
2k											
1k											

FITNESS TRACKER

Physical exercise is not only beneficial for the body, but it also enhances brain function. Yes, it makes your brain work better, and it releases endorphins in the brain that improve your mood and sense of well-being. Exercising, a positive coping strategy for dealing with stress, burns off adrenaline and improves sleep. Regular physical activity helps to prevent chronic diseases such as diabetes, obesity, depression, cancer, and heart disease.

Varying the types of fitness activity that you perform is beneficial. In the winter, I walk a couple of miles a week. But in the summer, I swim twenty laps in my pool twice a week. Bicycling is an excellent form of exercise to perform when it is hot outside.

I also have a vegetable garden and fruit orchard. I consider gardening and yard work a rigorous form of physical activity. You don't have to go to the gym to expend calories; you could just vacuum and mop the whole house. Therefore, I listed several different activities that I consider forms of fitness training.

Record the number of minutes you perform each activity on the following charts.

Day	Cardio	Strength	Group Fitness	Cleaning	Gardening
1					
2					
3					
4					
5					
6					
7					
8					
9					
10					
11					
12					
13					
14					
15					
16					
17					
18					
19					
20					
21					

And let us run with perseverance the race marked out for us, fixing
our eyes on Jesus, the pioneer and perfecter of faith.
Hebrews 12:1-2 (NIV)

Day	Cardio	Strength	Group Fitness	Cleaning	Gardening
22					
23					
24					
25					
26					
27					
28					
29					
30					
31					
32					
33					
34					
35					
36					
37					
38					
39					
40					
41					
42					

WEEKLY ENTRY INSTRUCTIONS

The first five days of each week include a devotion or educational snippet. However, the sixth and seventh days (Journal Time and Sabbath Reflections) are left blank to allow space for you to journal your thoughts, feelings, desires, and concerns.

Be sure to record daily information in the weekly Well-Being Chart and tracker tables for water, steps, and fitness. In addition, complete a Daily Food Journal provided at the end of each day's devotion.

As you experience:

- temptations—record this in the Temptation/Struggle log
- undesirable health issues—track these symptoms in the Issue Tracker
- binge—document the incident in the Binge Eating Tracker
- gratitude or victory—note this in the appropriate log
- new positive habits—record them in the New Healthy Living Habits Log
- defeat over temptation—write how you succeeded in

overcoming spiritually in Appendix 2: My Battle Strategies Plan
- other items not listed—track them in the Blank Log and Tracker

These logs and charts are at the beginning of this journal and the appendices in the back. Several pages are left blank for you to create your own log or tracker page.

Try not to be overwhelmed by the amount of entries as you begin this journal. Completing the process will only take a few minutes here and there each day, and the benefits of journaling will outweigh the time required.

17

DAILY FOOD JOURNAL
INSTRUCTIONS

This daily journal will appear after every day's devotion, so you understand how your food intake affects your overall well-being. Take the time each day to complete the chart so you can have a full picture of your journey to health and abundance.

The last three items at the bottom of the chart correspond to your symptoms after you ate. Add a Y for yes and N for no for those items. Recognize if there is a correlation between energy level, mental clarity, and mood after eating. Also, note whether you experienced any digestive discomfort.

After-Dinner Snack

Do not eat anything three hours before going to bed, and fast for twelve hours each night (from dinner until breakfast). This recommendation is for brain health, to prevent dementia and Alzheimer's. A clinical study that showed significant improvement in these diseases of the brain recommends these two interventions to reduce insulin levels.[2] Therefore, if you eat dinner at 7 p.m. and go to bed at 10 p.m., you should not eat a snack after dinner.

	Breakfast	Lunch	Snack	Dinner
Food				
Time				
Three Hours Since Last Meal?				
Hungry?				
Feel an Emotion? Describe:				
Satisfied or Stuffed				
Digestive Issue?				
Poor Mental Clarity?				
Bad Mood?				

PART I
WEEK 1

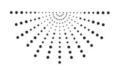

MENU PLAN

Planning my weekly menu takes about an hour, and I usually do this on Sunday. I list what I plan to cook for breakfast, lunch, dinner, and snack for every day of the week. As I choose a recipe, I put the ingredients I need on my corresponding grocery list.

After you create your menu and grocery list (subscribe to Susan-UNeal.com/healthy-living-blog for menus and lists), hit the grocery store or local farmer's market. Once your groceries are put away it is time to start cooking healthy homemade meals. Your body will appreciate your planning and food preparation, and being prepared will keep you from making unhealthy impulsive choices when you grocery shop.

Use the following chart to plan your weekly menu.

Meal	Monday	Tuesday
Breakfast		
Lunch		
Snack		
Dinner		

Meal	Wednesday	Thursday
Breakfast		
Lunch		
Snack		
Dinner		

Be sure to take the time needed each week to plan your menu. If you do, you will have healthy foods on hand and that will decrease the possibility of eating unhealthy meals and snacks.

Meal	Friday	Saturday
Breakfast		
Lunch		
Snack		
Dinner		

Meal	Sunday
Breakfast	
Lunch	
Snack	
Dinner	

WELL-BEING CHART

Determine how habits affect your well-being. Record the number of hours you slept and add a Y for yes and N for no for the other items tracked below. Recognize if there is a correlation between your energy level and mood with the consumption of unhealthy foods.

If you pay attention to your body and how it reacts to different types of food, you can figure out what items to eliminate from your diet. For me, it is anything with a high sugar content. I feel my body surge when I experience a sugar high; then it crashes as my blood-sugar level plummets. Afterward, I feel wiped out and devoid of energy. Unfortunately, the next day I suffer from brain fog and low energy.

When you figure out what food causes your body to react poorly, then you can avoid the food culprit. This is the puzzle you need to figure out. Through using this journal you will put the puzzle together.

Days	1	2	3	4	5	6	7
Hours of Sleep							
Ate Unhealthy Foods: List the foods							
Binged							
Low Energy Level							
Brain Fog							
Bad Mood							
Anxiety							
Irritable							
Digestive Issues							
Physical Activity							
Probiotics							
Spent Time w/ God							

Restful sleep is an essential component of a person's well-being. At least eight hours of sleep per night is recommended for optimal brain health and to prevent dementia and Alzheimer's.[1] These diseases of the brain are on the rise. Most everyone has a loved one or knows someone who suffers from one of these diseases. Your sleep and diet affect your brain. If you slept less than eight hours or consumed unhealthy foods, color the box red in the Well-Being Chart. If you experience a day with high energy and clarity of mind color the corresponding boxes green.

Many of the symptoms listed in the Well-Being Chart (energy, brain fog, mood, anxiety, irritability, digestive issues) are caused by the foods you consume. Recently, I noticed that home-made chocolate-chip cookies made with almond flour and maple syrup, although healthier, still made me irritable and less tolerant. My family does not deserve to be treated in an ill-tempered manner. Once I recognized the culprit, by journaling what I ate, I stopped snacking on the cookies.

Spending time with God can also affect your temperament. Most mornings I try to spend fifteen minutes of quiet, meditative time with the Lord. Getting connected with the Creator of the universe and feeling his presence in my life gives me a better sense of well-being. Asking for his help to maintain a healthy eating pattern gives me newfound strength.

Each week you will be provided with a new Well-Being Chart to complete on a daily basis. At the end of each week review your Daily Food Journal and compare it with your Well-Being Chart to determine how you did food wise along with the corresponding symptoms. When you color boxes red (negative symptoms) and green (positive symptoms) it is easier to figure out what type of food makes your body function well and what doesn't. When you find a food culprit, eliminate it from your diet.

DAY 1: INTRODUCTION

During the next six weeks, commit to spending a few minutes each day recording what you ate and drank and how your body reacted to those foods. Food issues you didn't know you had will become apparent because you can identify which items you ate that made you feel less than your best. For example, if I eat something that raises my blood sugar, the next day I experience brain fog and lethargy. How do you feel the day after consuming food with high sugar content? Write it down, and you will find out.

Each week's Daily Food Journal and Well-Being Chart will take you through what you should record. Tracking this information is important for your physical health, yet one of the most valuable components of journaling is recording what takes place in the mind. Understanding the emotional and spiritual implications you may have with food is essential to improving your lifestyle.

If you binge, what happens to your body? Write it down in the Binge Eating Log. Just as it is important to determine the nutritional content of food, it is vital to figure out the strongholds in your mind. A stronghold is something you turn to instead of God. Understanding your thoughts about food is necessary to determine the root cause of a dysfunctional food habit.

Recording thoughts, feelings, struggles, and victories has a powerful effect. Journaling also creates personal accountability. The more you journal, the more easily you'll recognize when you are eating out of emotion or for the wrong reason. You may determine what helped you overcome a struggle. Journaling provides clarity of thoughts, feelings, and desires.

If you need more guidance, I created the course, 7 Steps to Reclaim Your Health and Optimal Weight (SusanUNeal.com/courses/7-steps-to-get-off-sugar-and-carbs-course). This course will help you figure out and resolve the root cause of your inappropriate eating habits. One solved, taming your appetite is much easier. I show you how you can change your eating habits once and for all.

Are you living life to its fullness? Is your health or weight impeding you from embracing a healthy, abundant life? You are about to embark on the bountiful life Jesus has in store for you!

"The thief's purpose is to steal, kill and destroy. My purpose is to give life in all its fullness."

John 10:10 (TLB)

Father,

As I begin this journey to improve my health, help me find the time and motivation to record my thoughts and habits in this journal. Please guide me to reawaken the youth and vitality of the glorious body you gave me. Help me understand how different foods affect my body, so I can know if a specific food is harming me. Thank you in advance for helping me and answering my prayers. In Jesus's name. Amen.

	Breakfast	Lunch	Snack	Dinner
Food				
Time				
Three Hours Since Last Meal?				
Hungry?				
Feel an Emotion? Describe:				
Satisfied or Stuffed				
Digestive Issue?				
Poor Mental Clarity?				
Bad Mood?				

2

DAY 2: DECIDE TO IMPROVE YOUR HEALTH

I am delighted that you decided to reclaim your health. No one can force you to change; it has to be an internal motivation. Whether you are experiencing health issues, carrying excessive weight, or want to get your energy back, I am glad you are taking control of your well-being.

Through recording the information included in this journal, you will begin to solve a puzzle, one you couldn't figure out on your own. Each day you will discover a new piece of the puzzle as you understand what you need to do to improve your health. For example, you may not have been drinking enough water, so you experienced constipation. Or you drank half of your daily calories in a Starbucks Frappuccino, and this caused brain fog and fatigue.

As you uncover each new puzzle piece, you will discover how to make your body feel good again. As your energy improves, you will be motivated to go for a walk or attend a social event. Jesus wants you to live life in all its fullness, not in a worn-out, sick body. So let's get going and find out why you are experiencing ill health or excessive weight. Decide to enrich your lifestyle and record each day's information in this journal, so your health will improve.

Deciding is the first step to transformation. Begin by asking God to make you willing to change. Once you are willing, write down the changes you will make, and commit to them before the Lord. Include the measurable goals you would like to achieve in the Healthy Living Goals section at the beginning of this journal. Ask God to help you and place your success in his loving arms.

Write your commitment below:

Now state in a firm voice (speak out loud) the commitment you just made to God.

Crowds of sick people—blind, lame, or paralyzed—lay on the porches. One of the men lying there had been sick for thirty-eight years. When Jesus saw him and knew he had been ill for a long time, he asked him, "Would you like to get well?"

John 5:3–6

Dear Lord,

I want to feel and look good again. I know I have not always taken care of my body and I am sorry. Please help me do better. I want to serve and please you, and I can do that best if I am well. Help me discover why my body is not functioning the way you intended. In Jesus's name, I pray. Amen.

	Breakfast	Lunch	Snack	Dinner
Food				
Time				
Three Hours Since Last Meal?				
Hungry?				
Feel an Emotion? Describe:				
Satisfied or Stuffed				
Digestive Issue?				
Poor Mental Clarity?				
Bad Mood?				

3

DAY 3: HEALTHY EATING GUIDELINES

The following healthy eating guidelines are my secret to maintaining optimal weight and brain health. This is a low-carbohydrate, low-glycemic, anti-inflammatory eating plan, which is the type of diet recommended for improving memory and cognition and preventing and reversing type 2 diabetes. You can obtain a printable version of these Healthy Eating Guidelines at SusanUNeal.com/appendix (appendix 5 of *7 Steps to Get Off of Sugar and Carbohydrates*).

Low-carbohydrate, anti-inflammatory dietary guidelines include:

- About 50 percent of food items are fresh organic vegetables.
- Eat one fresh, raw serving of low-glycemic fruit per day. Low-glycemic fruits include green apples, berries, cherries, pears, plums, and grapefruit.
- Do not always eat cooked foods. Eat a couple of servings of raw vegetables every day. Have a salad for lunch with either nuts or meat. When eating out, order a salad or coleslaw as sides, since both are raw.
- Another 25 percent of your daily food intake should come

from an animal or vegetable protein such as beans, nuts, and lean meats. Fish is exceptionally nutritious. Try to eat it once a week.

- A variety of different nuts and seeds are excellent sources of protein, minerals, and essential fatty acids.

- Avoid sugar, flour, rice, pasta, and bread. Instead, eat more fruits, vegetables, and low-glycemic grains such as quinoa and pearled barley.

- Beware of GMO Roundup Ready crops (most oat, corn, wheat, beet, and soy in the United States) that may contain residue from the carcinogen glyphosate (active ingredient in Roundup).[3] Therefore, buy only organic oat, corn, wheat, beet, and soy products.

- Do not eat sugary cereals. Instead, eat oatmeal, fruit, or granola. Be careful, as the sugar content of granola may be high. My favorite granola recipe appears in appendix 4 of *7 Steps to Get Off Sugar and Carbohydrates*.

- Try not to eat anything containing more than 10 grams of sugar in one serving.

- Eat nontraditional grains such as quinoa, amaranth, pearled barley, wild rice, and organic oats.

- Eat cultured foods such as kimchi, sauerkraut, and cultured plain Greek yogurt since they contain natural probiotics. Add one to two tablespoons of these foods to a meal twice a week or eat the yogurt as a snack. Personally I take a probiotic capsule every day.

- Replace sugary snacks with nuts, nut butter, dark chocolate, and plain Greek yogurt with berries.

- Replace condiments and sauces containing MSG or high-fructose corn syrup with spices, vinegar, and herbs.

- Replace fried foods with baked foods.

My additional healthy eating tips include:

- Make homemade granola from organic oats. For breakfast, I add fresh berries to a bowl of granola.
- Buy or whip up a flavorful dip like hummus or guacamole to eat with a platter of fresh vegetables (not chips or pita bread).
- Substitute beans for meat for some meals.
- Squeeze a slice of lemon and two drops of stevia into a glass of water. It is like drinking fresh lemonade.
- Boil eggs and keep them in the refrigerator for a snack.
- Chew your food thoroughly because this is where digestion begins.

Please try not to be overwhelmed by all of this information. Guide your eating with the 80/20 percent rule. *If you eat healthy 80 percent of the time and not so healthy 20 percent of the time, this will probably be an improvement.* I don't eat perfectly, but I try. With God's help, I try to follow these healthy eating guidelines a large percentage of the time.

	Breakfast	Lunch	Snack	Dinner
Food				
Time				
Three Hours Since Last Meal?				
Hungry?				
Feel an Emotion? Describe:				
Satisfied or Stuffed				
Digestive Issue?				
Poor Mental Clarity?				
Bad Mood?				

4

DAY 4: HOW DIFFERENT FOODS AFFECT YOUR BODY

Each of us has a unique body that reacts differently to various foods. High sugar content in foods causes problems in my system. Someone else may react negatively to the large gluten molecule of today's modern hybridized wheat. If you want to find out if you are gluten sensitive, either fast from gluten for a whole month, or take the Gluten Quiz at GlutenIntoleranceQuiz.com.

The purpose of this journal is to help you become aware of how different foods affect your body. Evaluate every item before you eat it to determine whether it is beneficial for you. Then pay attention to how you feel after you eat a specific food. By doing this, you can figure out what causes digestive problems, sleep disturbances, allergies, etc.

This is not a weight-loss program but a lifestyle change to improve your overall health so you feel better and therefore can serve God (and your family) to the best of your ability. If you evaluate everything you eat and ask yourself, "Did God create this food or did a food manufacturer make it to fatten their bottom line?" then you will begin changing your eating choices.

Many times we ignore what our body is trying to tell us. Instead, pay attention to it. Don't shrug off a symptom. Notice it and document it in the Issue Tracker at the beginning of this journal.

For decades my sister had to be close to a bathroom the day after she ate an unbeknownst type of food. It was terrible to be on a vacation and not know when this issue would occur. The problem was that she was sensitive to gluten and did not know it. She suffered for many years but, had she used a journal like this one, she could have figured out the offending food .

What type of undesirable symptom do you experience? Would you like to alleviate the symptom? (Fill out the Issue Tracker every time you experience the symptom.)

_____

_____

	Breakfast	Lunch	Snack	Dinner
Food				
Time				
Three Hours Since Last Meal?				
Hungry?				
Feel an Emotion? Describe:				
Satisfied or Stuffed				
Digestive Issue?				
Poor Mental Clarity?				
Bad Mood?				

5

DAY 5: MENU PLANNING

During this six-week period set aside time every week to plan your menu and grocery list. If you don't, you may end up eating unhealthy foods because you didn't take time to prepare properly. If you would like menus, recipes, and corresponding grocery lists, subscribe to my blog at SusanUNeal.com/healthy-living-blog.

While grocery shopping, shop along the edges of the store in the produce and refrigerated sections. Stay away from the center of the store where processed foods experience an extended shelf life. Remember, a long shelf life means the nutritional value of the food has been removed. If a food spoils, it is beneficial to the human body, but if it does not spoil, it contains no nutrients. Food in boxes and bags do not benefit the body but harm it.

What boxed or bagged food items do you need to eliminate?

_____

. . .

What obstacles do you face in creating a weekly menu and shopping list? How can you address these challenges to start a new way of food planning?

_____

_____

_____

Who in your family can you enlist to help you in menu planning and/or shopping? How can they partner with you to help?

_____

_____

_____

	Breakfast	Lunch	Snack	Dinner
Food				
Time				
Three Hours Since Last Meal?				
Hungry?				
Feel an Emotion? Describe:				
Satisfied or Stuffed				
Digestive Issue?				
Poor Mental Clarity?				
Bad Mood?				

6

DAY 6: JOURNAL TIME

	Breakfast	Lunch	Snack	Dinner
Food				
Time				
Three Hours Since Last Meal?				
Hungry?				
Feel an Emotion? Describe:				
Satisfied or Stuffed				
Digestive Issue?				
Poor Mental Clarity?				
Bad Mood?				

7

DAY 7: SABBATH REFLECTIONS

	Breakfast	Lunch	Snack	Dinner
Food				
Time				
Three Hours Since Last Meal?				
Hungry?				
Feel an Emotion? Describe:				
Satisfied or Stuffed				
Digestive Issue?				
Poor Mental Clarity?				
Bad Mood?				

PART II
WEEK 2

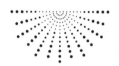

MENU PLAN

To ease the task of menu planning, I created a standard grocery list for the store I used. To create this list, initially I walked through the store and either wrote or dictated into my smartphone notes app the items I normally purchased on each grocery aisle. For example, I would start in the back of the store in the refrigerated section and would include eggs, butter, and coconut milk on the list for that aisle. Then I proceeded to the next aisle: cleaning supplies and paper products. I listed toilet paper, napkins, paper towels, paper plates, etc. And so on, until I compiled a master grocery.

At home, I typed out this list based on each grocery store aisle and the products I usually purchased. It took work to create this list, but it streamlined my grocery store planning for years.

Each week I printed a fresh new grocery list and my family knew that if we ran out of an item, they were supposed to circle it on the list or write it out. I made a rule to guide us—if it wasn't on the list, it didn't get purchased. I put the responsibility on them, not all on me.

Use the following chart to plan out your menu.

Meal	Monday	Tuesday
Breakfast		
Lunch		
Snack		
Dinner		

Meal	Wednesday	Thursday
Breakfast		
Lunch		
Snack		
Dinner		

Meal	Friday	Saturday
Breakfast		
Lunch		
Snack		
Dinner		

Meal	Sunday
Breakfast	
Lunch	
Snack	
Dinner	

WELL-BEING CHART

The following Well-Being Chart will help you determine how your habits affect your well-being. Record the number of hours you slept and add a Y for yes and N for no for the other items tracked below. Recognize if there is a correlation between your energy level and mood with the consumption of unhealthy foods. List those foods on the chart.

Your sleep and diet affect your brain. If you slept less than eight hours or ate unhealthy foods, color the box red in the Well-Being Chart. If you experience a day with high energy and clarity of mind color the corresponding boxes green.

Many of the symptoms listed in the Well-Being Chart (energy, brain fog, mood, anxiety, irritability, digestive issues) are affected by the foods you consume.

At the end of the week review your Daily Food Journals and compare it with your Well-Being Chart to determine how you did food wise along with the corresponding symptoms. When you color boxes red (negative symptoms) and green (positive symptoms) it is easier to figure out what type of food makes your body function well and vice-versa. When you find a food culprit, eliminate it from your diet.

Record the information below.

Days	8	9	10	11	12	13	14
Hours of Sleep							
Ate Unhealthy Foods: List the foods							
Binged							
Low Energy Level							
Brain Fog							
Bad Mood							
Anxiety							
Irritable							
Digestive Issues							
Physical Activity							
Probiotics							
Spent Time w/ God							

8

DAY 8: ACQUIRE KNOWLEDGE

Have you ever found yourself eating something you thought was nutritious, only to find out later it wasn't? In our society it is difficult to navigate diet trends. In the 1980s, low-fat diets were the trend; now the ketogenic diet is popular. However, these eating methods seem to be the exact opposite. Which one is best?

Lack of knowledge is a key reason people fall into the trap of unintentionally eating the wrong types of food. When people gain knowledge, they recognize that their previous beliefs were false, and it becomes easier to overcome unhealthy eating habits. Acquiring knowledge regarding unhealthy versus healthy foods is crucial to making this lifestyle change. If you are serious about improving your health and weight, follow the seven simple steps in *7 Steps to Get Off Sugar and Carbohydrates* (see Day 11: Seven-Step Plan).

When you apply God's wisdom, along with accurate knowledge about today's food, you will improve your health and weight. Once you have the knowledge you need to make the right decision for your health, you'll be better equipped to take the next step, and the next, until you've changed your lifestyle. With your lifestyle change, you will live the abundant life Jesus wants you to experience, not a life filled with disease and unwanted, unhealthy symptoms.

. . .

My people are destroyed from lack of knowledge.

Hosea 4:6 (NIV)

	Breakfast	Lunch	Snack	Dinner
Food				
Time				
Three Hours Since Last Meal?				
Hungry?				
Feel an Emotion? Describe:				
Satisfied or Stuffed				
Digestive Issue?				
Poor Mental Clarity?				
Bad Mood?				

9

DAY 9: FOOD ADDICTION

The overabundance of delicacies in our society is hard to resist. Regrettably, people become addicted to sugar and carbs to the point that it causes excessive weight gain or health issues.

Sugar triggers the release of dopamine in the brain, which is part of our bodies' feel-good reward system. We enjoy the feeling of dopamine, so we keep eating carbs. At some point, an overconsumption of sugar and processed food rewires the brain's neural pathways and causes a person to become addicted.

The brain's hijacking triggers binge eating despite its consequences of weight gain and health problems. Therefore, getting off sugar is more complex than it may seem. It is no longer about willpower and self-discipline but a *biochemical addiction*.

Determining whether you are a food addict will help you understand yourself and enable you to effectively overcome this addiction. Take an online quiz to determine if you are addicted to food, by going to SusanUNeal.com/Resources. If your test was positive, I recommend you do the study in *Christian Study Guide for 7 Steps to Get Off Sugar and Carbohydrates*.

. . .

Do you eat in a manner you do not like? If yes, how?

_____

_____

_____

Do you think you have a food addiction? Journal your thoughts here:

_____

_____

_____

If you have a food addiction, what have the consequences been for you?

_____

_____

_____

. . .

Similarly, Paul struggled as indicated in this scripture:

The trouble is with me, for I am all too human, a slave to sin. I don't really understand myself, for I want to do what is right, but I don't do it. Instead, I do what I hate.

Romans 7:14–15

Dear Lord,

I know many of the foods I consume are not beneficial for me, but I can't seem to change. Please help me figure out what is going on inside of my body so I can gain control. It is nice to know that Paul struggled to do "what is right." Help me Lord to do what is right and pleasing in your sight. Jesus, through your holy name, I pray. Amen.

	Breakfast	Lunch	Snack	Dinner
Food				
Time				
Three Hours Since Last Meal?				
Hungry?				
Feel an Emotion? Describe:				
Satisfied or Stuffed				
Digestive Issue?				
Poor Mental Clarity?				
Bad Mood?				

10

DAY 10: CANDIDA

God made the human gastrointestinal (GI) system with the perfect balance of beneficial microorganisms. However, when a person consumes the standard American diet containing dyes, chemicals, excess sugar, and the residue of pesticides and herbicides, it disrupts the gut's equilibrium. The primary offender of this imbalance is antibiotics. They kill the good microbes and thereby, cause a bad guy —Candida—to overgrow. Candida makes a person crave sugar, alcohol, wheat, and processed foods because that is what it eats.

Candida Albicans, a type of yeast common in the gut, can grow roots into the lining of your GI system. The fungal overgrowth can create openings in the bowel walls, which is known as a leaky gut. These holes allow harmful microorganisms to enter the bloodstream. Our bodies don't recognize these particles, so our immune system creates antibodies, which cause food allergies and autoimmune diseases to develop.[4] An overgrowth of Candida also causes the abdomen to become distended.

When Candida spreads out of control, it acts like a parasite sucking the life and energy out of you. It is like a monster growing inside of you, craving sugar, and it is hard to fight its ever-increasing appetite. I had an overgrowth of Candida, so I know how hard it is to fight this culprit.

If you want to determine if you have a candida overgrowth in your gut, take the Candida Quiz at CandiQuiz.com. In addition, to you could take a simple spit test. First thing in the morning, before you drink anything or brush your teeth, spit into a glass of water. In one to three minutes, check the cup to see if any strings hang down from the spit—strings are a positive sign of Candida. The spit will resemble a jellyfish. If the water becomes cloudy or the saliva sinks to the bottom, this is also a sign of Candida. Healthy saliva floats on the top of the water with no strings hanging down.

To kill the bug in your gut (Candida) take an anti-Candida cleanse. Read the instructions on the cleanse package for how to administer it. Initially, I recommend taking the cleanse every other day for the first week to minimize lethargy and headaches. You will feel awful if the dead Candida is not quickly expelled from your colon. To avoid becoming constipated, drink plenty of water and increase the fiber in your diet.

The first three days you are on the cleanse, you may not feel well, but after a week you will begin to feel better than you have in a long time. You are just about to get the life back Jesus wants you to experience—one that is abundant and full.

If you would like more specific instructions about getting rid of Candida, get a copy of *7 Steps to Get Off Sugar and Carbohydrates* so you can start your journey to optimal health.

	Breakfast	Lunch	Snack	Dinner
Food				
Time				
Three Hours Since Last Meal?				
Hungry?				
Feel an Emotion? Describe:				
Satisfied or Stuffed				
Digestive Issue?				
Poor Mental Clarity?				
Bad Mood?				

11

DAY 11: SEVEN-STEP PLAN

Would you like to improve the way you feel and look while increasing your energy level and clarity of mind? How about losing weight naturally without going on a fad diet or buying prepared meals and supplements? You can achieve these results by implementing the following seven steps.

Seven Steps to Get Off Sugar and Carbs

Step 1. Decide to improve your health through proper nutrition.

Step 2. Acquire a support system and knowledge to help make a lifestyle change.

Step 3. Clean out your pantry and refrigerator by removing unhealthy foods and clean out your emotions with God.

Step 4. Purchase healthy foods and an anti-Candida cleanse.

Step 5. Plan for the date to begin changing your eating habits and implement the following seven-day eating plan listed below.

Step 6. Prepare and eat foods differently than you did before.

Step 7. Improve your health through continuing this new lifestyle never turning back to your old eating habits.

. . .

Seven-Day Eating Plan

Day 1: Drink your recommended amount of water per day. Stop eating sugar. Take a probiotic.

Day 2: Stop eating wheat.

Day 3: Do not eat processed foods out of boxes and bags. Eat 50 percent of your food fresh and raw. Follow the Healthy Eating Guidelines provided in appendix 5 of *7 Steps to Get Off Sugar and Carbohydrates*. Obtain a printable version of this plan at SusanUNeal.com/appendix.

Days 4 and 5: Focus on you. Rest, read, pray, and ask God to give you the willpower to succeed.

Day 6: Begin the anti-Candida cleanse.

Day 7: Get up and exercise.

These seven steps were taken from *7 Steps to Get Off Sugar and Carbohydrates.*

What steps do you plan to initiate?

	Breakfast	Lunch	Snack	Dinner
Food				
Time				
Three Hours Since Last Meal?				
Hungry?				
Feel an Emotion? Describe:				
Satisfied or Stuffed				
Digestive Issue?				
Poor Mental Clarity?				
Bad Mood?				

DAY 12: FOODS TO ELIMINATE

Understanding what foods are beneficial versus harmful is confusing today, especially since the food industry entices us through great marketing strategies and by adding addictive ingredients. It is far better to eat foods as close to their value at harvest—the way God made them—rather than processed foods.

You should eliminate the following foods from your diet:

- wheat—hybridized and most humans can't digest the gluten
- white flour—stripped of its nutrients
- sugar—addictive and raises blood-sugar levels and predisposes a person to diabetes
- corn syrup, also called high-fructose corn syrup— inexpensive alternative to sugar with the same devastating effects
- white rice—stripped of its nutrients
- corn (except organic)—most are GMO Roundup Ready crops and may contain the carcinogen glyphosate
- milk products—denatured of its nutritional value to extend

its shelf life and since it doesn't contain its natural enzymes human beings cannot properly digest it

- artificial sweeteners—causes a person to crave sweets
- processed meats—the World Health Organization classified processed meats (hot dogs, ham, bacon, sausage, and some deli meats) as a group 1 carcinogen[5]
- vegetable oils except for coconut and olive oil—most vegetable oils contain omega 6 fatty acids, which promote inflammation in the human body
- processed foods contained in boxes and bags—the nutrients and fiber are removed to increase their shelf life
- canned goods—lined with Bisphenol (BPA), which is a hormone disruptor, prevent erosion of the can
- margarine—contains trans-fat, which increases the risk of heart disease, and free radicals, which contribute to numerous health problems including cancer
- sugar-sweetened drinks, fruit juices—addictive, raise blood-sugar levels, and predispose a person to diabetes

By reducing or eliminating these foods you will improve the health of your body. For a complete explanation as to why you should stop eating these foods, read Step 3: Clean Out the Pantry and Refrigerator of *7 Steps to Get Off Sugar and Carbohydrates*.

	Breakfast	Lunch	Snack	Dinner
Food				
Time				
Three Hours Since Last Meal?				
Hungry?				
Feel an Emotion? Describe:				
Satisfied or Stuffed				
Digestive Issue?				
Poor Mental Clarity?				
Bad Mood?				

13

DAY 13: JOURNAL TIME

	Breakfast	Lunch	Snack	Dinner
Food				
Time				
Three Hours Since Last Meal?				
Hungry?				
Feel an Emotion? Describe:				
Satisfied or Stuffed				
Digestive Issue?				
Poor Mental Clarity?				
Bad Mood?				

14

DAY 14: SABBATH REFLECTIONS

	Breakfast	Lunch	Snack	Dinner
Food				
Time				
Three Hours Since Last Meal?				
Hungry?				
Feel an Emotion? Describe:				
Satisfied or Stuffed				
Digestive Issue?				
Poor Mental Clarity?				
Bad Mood?				

PART III
WEEK 3

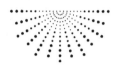

MENU PLAN

WEEKLY MENU PLANNING

This is an example of my cooking plan for a week. I cooked on Sunday and Monday and had leftovers (from Sunday) to be served on Tuesday. Wednesday we all ate at church, and Thursday I served leftovers from Monday. To liven up a leftover, I would cook one new item (such as a vegetable) to be served with the previous meal, and this new item gave the meal new interest. Two nights of cooking took care of four meals.

Every week I made a large, fresh, raw salad (broccoli salad, beet salad, cole slaw, salad with lettuce) and I ate that for my lunch throughout the week. I have over fifty recipes in the printable version of appendix 4 from *7 Steps to Get Off Sugar and Carbohydrates* at Susan-UNeal.com/appendix. For my children's lunch boxes, I tried to include one fresh fruit and vegetable each day.

Use the following chart to plan out your weekly menu.

Meal	Monday	Tuesday
Breakfast		
Lunch		
Snack		
Dinner		

Meal	Wednesday	Thursday
Breakfast		
Lunch		
Snack		
Dinner		

Meal	Friday	Saturday
Breakfast		
Lunch		
Snack		
Dinner		

Meal	Sunday
Breakfast	
Lunch	
Snack	
Dinner	

WELL-BEING CHART

The following Well-Being Chart will help you determine how your habits affect your well-being. Record the number of hours you slept and add a Y for yes and N for no for the other items tracked below. Recognize if there is a correlation between your energy level and mood with the consumption of unhealthy foods. List those foods on the chart.

Your sleep and diet affect your brain. If you slept less than eight hours or ate unhealthy foods, color the box red in the Well-Being Chart. If you experience a day with high energy and clarity of mind color the corresponding boxes green.

Many of the symptoms listed in the Well-Being Chart (energy, brain fog, mood, anxiety, irritability, digestive issues) are affected by the foods you consume.

At the end of the week review your Daily Food Journals and compare it with your Well-Being Chart to determine how you did food wise along with the corresponding symptoms. When you color boxes red (negative symptoms) and green (positive symptoms) it is easier to figure out what type of food makes your body function well and vice-versa. When you find a food culprit, eliminate it from your diet.

Please complete the information below.

Days	15	16	17	18	19	20	21
Hours of Sleep							
Ate Unhealthy Foods: List the foods							
Binged							
Low Energy Level							
Brain Fog							
Bad Mood							
Anxiety							
Irritable							
Digestive Issues							
Physical Activity							
Probiotics							
Spent Time w/ God							

15

DAY 15: ACCOUNTABILITY/PRAYER PARTNER

Acquiring a support system is integral to attaining success as you change your lifestyle. Therefore, ask someone to be your accountability and prayer partner. But first pray and ask God to give you wisdom to choose the right person.

That person should be someone who can understand the struggles you face but will not merely give you platitudes or think you should be able to "just do it." Your accountability partner should be one who will not give you permission to keep up your bad habits but will be both empathetic and truthful with you. Also, make sure this person is a Christian, so they can give you biblical advice and feel comfortable praying with you.

When someone understands how you feel, you are validated in your struggles, so it is helpful to reach out to a friend during this journey. Having a friend for accountability whom you can call when temptation arises is key to your success. It is powerful when someone speaks the truth in love.

Pray with your friend. The security of knowing this person prays for you is comforting. The following scripture confirms we should share trials and confess our sins to one another.

· · ·

Confess your sins to each other and pray for each other so that you may be healed.

James 5:16

Dear heavenly Father,

Please help me to find the perfect prayer and accountability partner—one whom I can open up to and share my thoughts, struggles, and feelings. Thank you, Lord. Through Jesus's name I pray. Amen.

Who are you going to ask to be your accountability/prayer partner? When do you plan to ask this person?

_____

_____

What other type of support would be beneficial?

_____

_____

_____

	Breakfast	Lunch	Snack	Dinner
Food				
Time				
Three Hours Since Last Meal?				
Hungry?				
Feel an Emotion? Describe:				
Satisfied or Stuffed				
Digestive Issue?				
Poor Mental Clarity?				
Bad Mood?				

16

DAY 16: TEMPTATION AND THE SWORD OF THE SPIRIT

When it comes to food, each of us struggles with temptation. I tend to overindulge with popcorn. While watching a movie, slowly but surely the whole tub disappears. So it is better for me to purchase a smaller portion. That's how I handle my temptation. You also need to figure out how to handle your food temptation.

What food struggle did you experience recently and how did you handle it? What would you do differently?

. . .

What time of day do you experience the most temptation?

Where were you when you were most tempted?

Was anyone with you when you were tempted?

Did you experience a strong emotion before you ate an unhealthy food? If yes, what was the feeling? Have you experienced this before?

. . .

As you figure out how to fight food temptation, record your strategies in Appendix 2: My Battle Strategies Plan. Then refer back to them as needed.

Sword of the Spirit

One of the ways to fight food addiction is through scripture. Appendix 1 of *7 Steps to Get Off Sugar and Carbohydrates* includes Bible verses to recite to tap into God's power and strength. You can obtain a printable version of this appendix at SusanUNeal.com/appendix. If you are addicted to sugar and carbohydrates, you need God's superpower.

Find a specific Bible verse to oppose your food issue and write it on an index card. Keep it with you until you memorize it. Speak the verse out loud every time you feel the urge to eat unhealthy foods.

When you choose to learn God's Word it will affect you positively in ways you can't imagine. We are supposed to store his word in our hearts. If we do we can draw upon them when the enemy whispers lies. Store the sword of the Spirit in your mind, so you can defeat Satan, and successfully achieve your goals.

I have hidden your word in my heart
   that I might not sin against you.

Psalm 119:11

Choose your strategic Bible verse and write it here. It is your sword; carry it with you and unsheathe it as needed.

. . .

	Breakfast	Lunch	Snack	Dinner
Food				
Time				
Three Hours Since Last Meal?				
Hungry?				
Feel an Emotion? Describe:				
Satisfied or Stuffed				
Digestive Issue?				
Poor Mental Clarity?				
Bad Mood?				

17

DAY 17: PRAYER

Prayer is an essential component of the arsenal God gave us, as Paul indicated in Ephesians 6:18, "And pray in the Spirit on all occasions with all kinds of prayers and requests" (NIV). To make the lifestyle changes necessary to improve your health, access your heavenly father through prayer. Prayer breaks down the resistance you may experience as you make these changes.

When Jesus was in Gethsemane, he prayed to his Father. We need to follow Jesus's example. God wants to communicate with us, and through prayer we receive his power to face our struggles. Ask God to give you a willing spirit to surrender to him, and replace your desire for food with the desire to please and serve him.

Jesus's brother told us:

The earnest prayer of a righteous man has great power and wonderful results.

James 5:16 (TLB)

Spend a few minutes telling God how you feel and what you desire. Ask him to help you achieve your goals. Tell him about your disappointments, and ask him to empower you during your struggles.

	Breakfast	Lunch	Snack	Dinner
Food				
Time				
Three Hours Since Last Meal?				
Hungry?				
Feel an Emotion? Describe:				
Satisfied or Stuffed				
Digestive Issue?				
Poor Mental Clarity?				
Bad Mood?				

18

DAY 18: MEDITATING WITH GOD

Most mornings I sit in the living room with my cup of tea and spend time with God. I close my eyes and focus on the Lord. While I draw in a deep breath, my mind drifts. Situations I didn't realize were significant to me become apparent. Emotions I suppressed resurface. The Lord purges and percolates my whole being to reveal what's truly important. Spending a few minutes every morning with him brings peace to my mind and soul.

Christian meditation is beneficial to our overall well-being. Mindfulness exercises such as Christian yoga train a person's mind to pay attention to cravings without reacting to them. When a person becomes more mindful, she notices why she wants to indulge but can move through the feeling without reacting to it. I created several Christian yoga products including DVDs, books, and card decks, available at ChristianYoga.com, which could help you become more mindful.

I will meditate about your glory, splendor, majesty, and miracles.

Psalm 145:5 (TLB)

Meditate on the Lord and journal your thoughts.

_____

_____

_____

_____

_____

_____

_____

_____

	Breakfast	Lunch	Snack	Dinner
Food				
Time				
Three Hours Since Last Meal?				
Hungry?				
Feel an Emotion? Describe:				
Satisfied or Stuffed				
Digestive Issue?				
Poor Mental Clarity?				
Bad Mood?				

19

DAY 19: FIVE-STEPS TO FREEDOM FROM ADDICTION

If you are addicted to food, you can gain freedom by implementing the five steps in the plan below. You can obtain a printable version of this plan from appendix 8 in *7 Steps to Get Off Sugar and Carbohydrates* by going to SusanUNeal.com/appendix. Post the five-step plan on your refrigerator or bathroom mirror and use it when tempted to overeat unhealthy foods.

1. Name what controls you.

Name the thing controlling you—food addiction, anxiety, eating disorder, depression, etc.—whatever it may be, and declare (out loud) Jesus Christ is your Lord in its place![6]

Stand up to the evil spirit who brought bondage into your life by saying, "Evil spirit, you won't lord over me or entice me through (insert your addiction) anymore. Jesus is my Lord!" A person obtains spiritual power and authority through Christ. Declare that the spiritual powers of darkness will not have lordship over your life. They will not rule you, govern your behavior, capture your thought life, or lead you into temptation and sin because "the one who is in you is greater than the one who is in the world" (1 John 4:4 NIV).

. . .

2. Submit yourself completely to God.

"Submit yourself, then, to God. Resist the devil, and he will flee from you." James 4:7 (NIV)

There is a secret to resisting the devil—you must first submit yourself to God. How in the world do you do that? In my experience, you no longer do your will but God's will by submitting your life to him.

3. Use the name of Jesus.

In the book of Acts, the apostles healed and worked miracles in the name of Jesus. Use Jesus's name as Peter did in Acts 3:6: "In the name of Jesus Christ of Nazareth, *walk!*" (TLB). Using the name of Jesus is key to binding the spiritual nature of an addiction, because then you operate under Jesus's authority.

4. Use the Word of God.

The Holy Spirit inside of you is stronger than Satan and his demons. By using the name of Jesus, you are not only under his authority but you can speak with his authority. You are much better armed than Satan. Now is the time to stand up to him, strip him of his weapons, and kick him out of your life through the Word of God! Speak out loud, "In the name of Jesus, you won't oppress me anymore. I bind your power in the name of Jesus and by the Word of God."

5. Praise God and practice gratitude.

When you praise God and thank him for his blessings, the demonic forces won't hang around. Fill your mind, heart, and body with the Spirit of God by putting the right things in your spirit. Listen to praise music; read the Bible and pray; memorize scripture; attend church, Sunday school, or a Bible study. Also start doing more to help others. Performing acts of service and helping others fills your heart with honorable feelings and humility. Every day write in your journal about all you can praise God for and thank him.

Beat the addiction by declaring Bible verses out loud. Stomp the spiritual nature of the addiction into the ground by singing praises to God. The devil can't stand to be around someone who worships the Lord. Become God's warrior by using his mighty unseen weapons. Paul advises:

It is true that I am an ordinary, weak human being, but I don't use human plans and methods to win my battles. I use God's mighty weapons, not those made by men, to knock down the devil's strongholds.

2 Corinthians 10:3–4 (TLB)

You are God's mighty conqueror!

How do you intend to put this plan into action?

	Breakfast	Lunch	Snack	Dinner
Food				
Time				
Three Hours Since Last Meal?				
Hungry?				
Feel an Emotion? Describe:				
Satisfied or Stuffed				
Digestive Issue?				
Poor Mental Clarity?				
Bad Mood?				

20

DAY 20: JOURNAL TIME

	Breakfast	Lunch	Snack	Dinner
Food				
Time				
Three Hours Since Last Meal?				
Hungry?				
Feel an Emotion? Describe:				
Satisfied or Stuffed				
Digestive Issue?				
Poor Mental Clarity?				
Bad Mood?				

21

DAY 21: SABBATH REFLECTIONS

	Breakfast	Lunch	Snack	Dinner
Food				
Time				
Three Hours Since Last Meal?				
Hungry?				
Feel an Emotion? Describe:				
Satisfied or Stuffed				
Digestive Issue?				
Poor Mental Clarity?				
Bad Mood?				

PART IV
WEEK 4

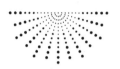

MENU PLAN

WEEKLY MENU PLANNING

Think of foods as being dead or alive. Food from a bag sitting on the shelf for months is dead and does not give your body any of the nutrients it needs to be healthy. A fresh piece of fruit contains essential vitamins, minerals, and fiber that the human body needs.

The fiber in fruits and vegetables you consume fills your stomach and tells your body you are full. When the fiber is removed, as in processed foods, it takes a larger quantity of food to become full. Also, the fiber in fruit slows digestion, which reduces the effects of sugar in raising your blood-sugar levels. As you eliminate processed foods from you diet you should consume more whole, organic fruits, vegetables, whole grains (oats, brown rice, quinoa, barley), beans, fish, and meat. Your body will thank you for nourishing it properly and will respond by healing itself.

Today, I look at any food and assess whether or not it is good for me. If a person primarily eats dead food, how does the body get the proper nutrients it needs? How can your body replace old cells with healthy new ones if you don't give it the essential vitamins and minerals it requires? If the body does not receive proper nutrition to perform the functions required for life and regeneration, it will break down. If cells within the human body replicate incorrectly cancer will develop.

Use the following chart to plan out your weekly menu.

Meal	Monday	Tuesday
Breakfast		
Lunch		
Snack		
Dinner		

Meal	Wednesday	Thursday
Breakfast		
Lunch		
Snack		
Dinner		

Meal	Friday	Saturday
Breakfast		
Lunch		
Snack		
Dinner		

Meal	Sunday
Breakfast	
Lunch	
Snack	
Dinner	

WELL-BEING CHART

The following Well-Being Chart will help you determine how habits affect your well-being. Record the number of hours you slept and add a Y for yes and N for no for the other items tracked below. Recognize if there is a correlation between your energy level and mood with the consumption of unhealthy foods. List those foods on the chart.

Your sleep and diet affect your brain. If you slept less than eight hours or ate unhealthy foods, color the box red in the Well-Being Chart. If you experience a day with high energy and clarity of mind color the corresponding boxes green.

Many of the symptoms listed in the Well-Being Chart (energy, brain fog, mood, anxiety, irritability, digestive issues) are affected by the foods you consume.

At the end of the week review your Daily Food Journals and compare it with your Well-Being Chart to determine how you did food wise along with the corresponding symptoms. When you color boxes red (negative symptoms) and green (positive symptoms) it is easier to figure out what type of food makes your body function well and vice-versa. When you find a food culprit, eliminate it from your diet.

Please complete the information below.

Days	22	23	24	25	26	27	28
Hours of Sleep							
Ate Unhealthy Foods: List the foods							
Binged							
Low Energy Level							
Brain Fog							
Bad Mood							
Anxiety							
Irritable							
Digestive Issues							
Physical Activity							
Probiotics							
Spent Time w/ God							

22

DAY 22: EMOTIONAL ISSUES WITH FOOD

For most of us, food and emotions are intrinsically tied together, so we need to do an emotional assessment and identify whether food brings us comfort.

If you need additional support figuring out emotional eating and how to resolve it, purchase my course, 7 Steps to Reclaim Your Health and Optimal Weight (https://susanuneal.com/courses/7-steps-to-get-off-sugar-and-carbs-course). In this course I walk you through the steps to change your eating habits once and for all.

How do you look at food? Are you using food to comfort yourself or meet an emotional need, or do you think of food as a necessity to keep your body functioning?

_____

_____

Do you turn to food to help you deal with life's challenges?

. . .

God gave us food to nourish our bodies. Yet food can be used for the wrong reasons. We may eat because we are sad, bored, stressed out, depressed, or happy. As we engage in emotional eating, we turn to food, instead of God, to appease ourselves. If we feel abandoned, food can be our friend. We can swallow our angry feelings with food, instead of feeling the emotions we don't want to deal with. Food can provide an emotional escape from negative feelings.

Do you use food to escape from emotional issues? If yes, how?

In your Daily Food Journal chart there is a column to document if you ate because you were hungry and if three hours passed since your last meal. On average it takes two to three hours for your previous meal to digest unless you ate fruit only. Each day determine if you are eating because of hunger or for some other reason. If you are not hungry, document why you are eating.

Do you have a deep emotional wound that needs healing? If you do, journal and talk to God about it. Is there someone you need to forgive? Maybe you have a big hole in your heart that you are filling with food.

God is our ultimate healer, take your wounds to him and ask him to heal you.

If you have an emotional connection with food, please consider using the *Christian Study Guide for 7 Steps to Get Off Sugar and Carbohydrates.* Whether you do this study by yourself or with a group, it will help you go more in-depth to resolve emotional issues once and for all. Please join my closed Facebook group, 7 Steps to Get Off Sugar, Carbs, and Gluten and share with me how you are doing. If you would like healthy living tips please like my Facebook page at Facebook.com/HealthyLivingSeries/.

Your weight does not determine your value to God. Your body is the temple of the Holy Spirit. Call on the Holy Spirit to empower you to change. With God's help, you can overcome and succeed.

The eyes of the LORD search the whole earth in order to strengthen those whose hearts are fully committed to him.

2 Chronicles 16:9

Dear Lord,

Please help me to understand my emotional connection with food. I want to replace my appetite with a desire for you. Please fill me with your Spirit and strengthen me. Turning to you first is what I want to do. Jesus, through your name, I pray. Amen.

	Breakfast	Lunch	Snack	Dinner
Food				
Time				
Three Hours Since Last Meal?				
Hungry?				
Feel an Emotion? Describe:				
Satisfied or Stuffed				
Digestive Issue?				
Poor Mental Clarity?				
Bad Mood?				

23

DAY 23: CLEAN OUT YOUR EMOTIONS

In this journal, record your thoughts as they relate to your consumption of food. The last two days of every week's devotions provide blank pages for you to write on. Figure out what triggers you to eat (when you are not hungry) and journal when you eat because of a negative emotion. This may help you identify dysfunctional eating behaviors.

What food problems have been with you since childhood? Take some time with God and record what instances from your past resulted in the way you eat today.

. . .

After you pinpoint your food issue, bring it to God and be honest with him about what you experience. Each time you recognize that you engage in emotional eating, clean out your emotions with the Lord so you can disengage the connection between eating and feelings.

Begin the process of cleaning out your emotions by telling God what you think is the origin of your unhealthy eating habit and ask him to help you heal from any emotional scars.

Changing your eating habits is not an overnight process. The more extended the period of unhealthy eating, the longer it will take to reset your body and mind. But step-by-step you can reprogram your body, mind, and spirit. Creating a support system and journaling are vital components to your success. You are on the path to recover your health and weight!

	Breakfast	Lunch	Snack	Dinner
Food				
Time				
Three Hours Since Last Meal?				
Hungry?				
Feel an Emotion? Describe:				
Satisfied or Stuffed				
Digestive Issue?				
Poor Mental Clarity?				
Bad Mood?				

24

DAY 24: BOREDOM/STRESS EATING

Sometimes we engage in mindless eating, where we munch on something without being hungry (for me it's popcorn). When a person is bored, she may look in the refrigerator or pantry but can't find anything appealing. If this happens to you, food is not what you need. First, drink two glasses of water, as you may be thirsty and don't realize it. Next, your soul may be longing for a connection with God, so spend time with him.

Journal your thoughts here.

· · ·

Stress also causes a person to turn to food. Determine the stressors (things that cause you stress) in your life. Can you do something about the stressors? Pray to God and ask him to enlighten you. Ask your accountability partner or support group for help and prayer in dealing with your stressors.

How do you cope with stress? Do you tend to deal with it through undesirable eating habits? If so, recognize this and choose to do something about your stress level. Some stress-relieving activities include getting a massage, journaling, calling a friend, and watching a movie.

Don't worry about anything; instead, pray about everything. Tell God what you need, and thank him for all he has done. Then you will experience God's peace, which exceeds anything we can understand. His peace will guard your hearts and minds as you live in Christ Jesus.

Philippians 4:6–7

I created an equation to correspond with this verse: Don't worry + Pray + Thank God + Abide in Jesus = God's Peace. Ask God to help you not worry, pray, thank him, and abide in Jesus so you can experience his peace that transcends all understanding.

Lord,

I need your help to stop worrying. Help me to turn to you and pray instead of turning to worldly things like food. I want to remember to thank you for even the small things. But most of all give me faith to believe Jesus is with me and I can call on him at any time to give me strength to overcome my battle with food. Thank you in advance for answering my prayer. Through Jesus's holy and precious name, I pray. Amen.

	Breakfast	Lunch	Snack	Dinner
Food				
Time				
Three Hours Since Last Meal?				
Hungry?				
Feel an Emotion? Describe:				
Satisfied or Stuffed				
Digestive Issue?				
Poor Mental Clarity?				
Bad Mood?				

DAY 25: BINGING

Overeating is unhealthy, and when that becomes a habit, eventually a person becomes addicted to food and can't stop eating it. In turn, this causes binging. Binge eating occurs when you can't stop eating an item even though you want to. You can't control yourself. Afterward, you regret what you did. If you binge, be sure to journal afterward in the Binge Eating Tracker. Determine your feelings before you binged and what temptation led you down that path.

Figure out your trigger and record it in the Temptation/Struggle Log. When you understand what tempts you, you can learn to avoid it.

What did you tell yourself that validated why it was okay to overeat?

. . .

Ask God to help you not to overindulge to the point of gluttony.

After binging, ask God to forgive you and help you not to binge again. Record your experience in the blank pages of the sixth or seventh day of each week's journal. Once you ask for forgiveness, God chooses not to remember your sins, as indicated in Hebrews 8:12: "And I will be merciful to them in their wrongdoings, and I will remember their sins no more" (TLB). Don't fret over a stumble. Get up and try again using the Five Spiritual Steps to Freedom from Addiction (day 19). You can get a printable copy of this plan at SusanUNeal.com/appendix; it is also in appendix 8 from *7 Steps to Get Off Sugar and Carbohydrates*.

If you record every incident of overeating in the Binge Eating Tracker and implement the five-step plan every time you binge, you will overcome and experience success. Retraining your mind is like disciplining a child; consistency is vital to transformation.

Don't copy the behavior and customs of this world, but let God transform you into a new person by changing the way you think. Then you will learn to know God's will for you, which is good and pleasing and perfect.

Romans 12:2

Father, Please transform me by changing the way I think. I need your power to beat this addiction to food. I can't do this without your transforming power, so I surrender my addiction to you. I believe you will instill your strength in me to meet this challenge so I can overcome it. I will replace my desire for food with your "pleasing and perfect" plan for me. Please remind me to seek you first and not food. Through Jesus's name I pray. Amen.

	Breakfast	Lunch	Snack	Dinner
Food				
Time				
Three Hours Since Last Meal?				
Hungry?				
Feel an Emotion? Describe:				
Satisfied or Stuffed				
Digestive Issue?				
Poor Mental Clarity?				
Bad Mood?				

26

DAY 26: FIGHT FOOD TEMPTATION

Every morning, first spend time with God. Then plan your day by determining your menu and what food struggles you might encounter. Decide how you will fight food temptation. Select a scripture verse to help you resist, and begin the day by reciting it out loud.

When you recognize temptation, remove yourself from the area containing the food, and record the enticement in the Temptation/Struggle Log at the beginning of this journal. Some strategies for resisting temptation include:

- pray
- go for a walk
- recite your Bible verse
- call your prayer partner
- drink two glasses of water
- listen to praise music and worship God
- spend time with and meditate about God

Record other helpful strategies you develop in Appendix 2: My Battle Strategies Plan. For a list of Food Addiction Battle Strategies, see appendix 1. Also, when you are tempted, think about how far you have come in overcoming your food addiction and whether you want to experience the withdrawal symptoms again.

Write down five reasons why you do not want to eat unhealthy food.

"And call on me in the day of trouble;
   I will deliver you, and you will honor me."

Psalm 50:15 (NIV)

Dear Lord,

Help me to plan my day, spend time with you, and successfully fight any food temptation I may encounter today. Jesus, give me strength. In your name I pray. Amen.

	Breakfast	Lunch	Snack	Dinner
Food				
Time				
Three Hours Since Last Meal?				
Hungry?				
Feel an Emotion? Describe:				
Satisfied or Stuffed				
Digestive Issue?				
Poor Mental Clarity?				
Bad Mood?				

27

DAY 27: JOURNAL TIME

	Breakfast	Lunch	Snack	Dinner
Food				
Time				
Three Hours Since Last Meal?				
Hungry?				
Feel an Emotion? Describe:				
Satisfied or Stuffed				
Digestive Issue?				
Poor Mental Clarity?				
Bad Mood?				

28

DAY 28: SABBATH REFLECTIONS

	Breakfast	Lunch	Snack	Dinner
Food				
Time				
Three Hours Since Last Meal?				
Hungry?				
Feel an Emotion? Describe:				
Satisfied or Stuffed				
Digestive Issue?				
Poor Mental Clarity?				
Bad Mood?				

PART V
WEEK 5

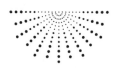

MENU PLAN

WEEKLY MENU PLANNING

Meals don't have to be complex. It wasn't complicated for Adam and Eve in the garden of Eden. They picked a piece of fruit or a vegetable and ate it. It doesn't have to be difficult for us either. Instead of making an elaborate meal, eat fresh, raw vegetables, which cost less and are better for you than processed, sugar-laden products.

Farmer's markets are great venues to find fresh, local produce. It is best to eat locally grown fruit and vegetables. Buy a potato and bake it with the following toppings: olive oil, broccoli, scallions, and sea salt with kelp (seaweed). The baked potato is better for you than a bag of potato chips. Eat foods closer to the form they were in when they came out of the garden.

Check labels and try not to eat foods with more than five ingredients and 10 grams of sugar per serving. The American Heart Association recommends you limit your calories from sugar to no more than half of your total calories, which is a lot. For most women in the US that should be no more than 24 grams of sugar or 100 calories per day. For men it is 36 grams of sugar or 150 calories from sugar per day.

If you can't pronounce an ingredient, your body probably won't recognize it as food either. Begin to simplify the foods you consume.

For example, eat two hard-boiled eggs for breakfast, a whole avocado for lunch, and an apple for a snack. Ask yourself, "Did the food I am about to eat exist in the garden of Eden?" Food doesn't have to be complicated.

Meal	Monday	Tuesday
Breakfast		
Lunch		
Snack		
Dinner		

Meal	Wednesday	Thursday
Breakfast		
Lunch		
Snack		
Dinner		

Meal	Friday	Saturday
Breakfast		
Lunch		
Snack		
Dinner		

Meal	Sunday
Breakfast	
Lunch	
Snack	
Dinner	

WELL-BEING CHART

The following Well-Being Chart will help you determine how habits affect your well-being. Record the number of hours you slept and add a Y for yes and N for no for the other items tracked below. Recognize if there is a correlation between your energy level and mood with the consumption of unhealthy foods. List those foods on the chart.

Your sleep and diet affect your brain. If you slept less than eight hours or ate unhealthy foods, color the box red in the Well-Being Chart. If you experience a day with high energy and clarity of mind color the corresponding boxes green.

Many of the symptoms listed in the Well-Being Chart (energy, brain fog, mood, anxiety, irritability, digestive issues) are affected by the foods you consume.

At the end of the week review your Daily Food Journals and compare it with your Well-Being Chart to determine how you did food wise along with the corresponding symptoms. When you color boxes red (negative symptoms) and green (positive symptoms) it is easier to figure out what type of food makes your body function well and vice-versa. When you find a food culprit, eliminate it from your diet.

Please complete the information below.

Days	29	30	31	32	33	34	35
Hours of Sleep							
Ate Unhealthy Foods: List the foods							
Binged							
Low Energy Level							
Brain Fog							
Bad Mood							
Anxiety							
Irritable							
Digestive Issues							
Physical Activity							
Probiotics							
Spent Time w/ God							

29

DAY 29: DIGESTIVE ISSUES

It is essential to notice how your body reacts to different foods. If you experience digestive problems, keep track of what you ate before the symptom—in the Issue Tracker at the beginning of this journal. Notice if you consistently belch after a particular type of food. If you do you may need to avoid this food or take a digestive enzyme (from a health food store). As we age or damage our GI tract, a person may not secrete enough digestive enzymes to break down their food properly. However, you can take an enzyme when you eat food so it will be digested properly.

Note whether you have problems digesting wheat or dairy, as these two products are the usual offenders. My culprit was sunflower and sesame seeds. I normally added those seeds to my homemade granola, but I often belched after I ate the granola. When I documented what I ate, I figured out what caused the digestive issue. When I eliminated those seeds from the recipe, my indigestion ceased.

Today's wheat is hybridized to the point that the gluten molecule is so large most humans cannot digest it. Therefore it is a major digestive offender. If you need to take an antacid, I recommend you stop eating wheat and see if your symptoms disappear.

· · ·

What type of digestive issues do you experience?

_____

	Breakfast	Lunch	Snack	Dinner
Food				
Time				
Three Hours Since Last Meal?				
Hungry?				
Feel an Emotion? Describe:				
Satisfied or Stuffed				
Digestive Issue?				
Poor Mental Clarity?				
Bad Mood?				

30

DAY 30: FOODS THAT CAUSE INFLAMMATION

Some medical literature claims inflammation is the root of chronic disease. Where do you think inflammation comes from? It generates from what we put into our bodies and most likely from food.

We eat many foods that are far from the products they were when first harvested. The human body does not recognize some of these so-called foods and so it reacts negatively and causes inflammation. Inflammation causes a wide-range of adverse effects across many systems in the body. It is critical to identify what food is causing a negative reaction in your body.

This journal will help you figure out this part of the puzzle. When you experience a negative physical symptom, record it in the Issue Tracker. Also note what foods you ate within the past twelve hours. You may recognize a pattern regarding a specific type of food. For me it was dairy; this food always caused me to experience congestion and postnasal drip at night.

If you think a specific food may be causing problematic symptoms in your body, eliminate it for at least a week. When you reintroduce it, be sure to record in your journal what symptoms you experience. If you would like me to coach you during this process, I am a Health and

Wellness Coach and I offer services at SusanUNeal.com/Health-Coaching.

What foods do you think may be causing you a problem?

_____

	Breakfast	Lunch	Snack	Dinner
Food				
Time				
Three Hours Since Last Meal?				
Hungry?				
Feel an Emotion? Describe:				
Satisfied or Stuffed				
Digestive Issue?				
Poor Mental Clarity?				
Bad Mood?				

31

DAY 31: FOOD SUBSTITUTES

As you begin to improve your eating habits, you need to find food substitutes. Many unhealthy food choices can be replaced with healthy alternatives that are whole, unprocessed, and natural. Here is a list of suggestions.

Sugar Substitutes
In the following list the best natural sugar substitutes are ranked based on their glycemic index:
stevia-0
monk fruit sweetener-0
xylitol-12
agave-15
coconut sugar-35
honey-50
maple syrup-54

Choose a natural, low-glycemic sweetener that you can live with and use it sparingly.

. . .

Pasta Substitutes

Cook spaghetti squash, shirataki, quinoa or chickpea noodles, or spiralize zucchini.

Milk Substitutes

It is best not to consume milk products. However, several healthy dairy substitutes include almond, cashew, coconut, and pea milk. I enjoy the flavor of toasted coconut almond blend, which combines both of these kinds of milk.

Which sugar, milk, or pasta substitute listed above will you commit to try?

_____

What type of foods have you eliminated so far? What food do you want to eliminate?

_____

Pray and ask God to give you the motivation and strength to make a positive lifestyle changes.

_____

. . .

_____

_____

	Breakfast	Lunch	Snack	Dinner
Food				
Time				
Three Hours Since Last Meal?				
Hungry?				
Feel an Emotion? Describe:				
Satisfied or Stuffed				
Digestive Issue?				
Poor Mental Clarity?				
Bad Mood?				

DAY 32: TIPS FOR A HEALTHIER LIFESTYLE

Simple changes like drinking plenty of water or eating only until you are full will help you transition into this new way of eating. Suggestions for choosing healthy foods when eating out are always needed. The following tips should assist you to successfully make healthy lifestyle changes.

Only Eat Until You're Full

As you prepare to eat healthier, one positive change you can make is to pay attention to the sensation of fullness as you eat. Some individuals may not be in touch with that feeling anymore. Focus on recognizing when you are full so you do not overeat. You may have to change some of your mealtime habits as well. Eat slowly, chew your food thoroughly, and pay attention to how the food tastes.

When you eat processed foods, versus meals you prepare from scratch, it takes a larger quantity of the refined product to fill your stomach because these foods do not contain the original food's fiber. Think of crushing a bag of chips versus shredding carrots and celery. The fresh vegetables will satiate your hunger with a smaller volume.

When you eat foods closer to their form at harvest, you will become full with smaller portions. The feeling of fullness stays with you for a longer period too, so you don't need to snack as much. By following this simple lifestyle change, you will eat a smaller quantity of food loaded with vitamins, minerals, fiber, and all the nutrients the human body needs—the way God intended for you to eat.

Pay attention to portion size. Think of your stomach as the size of your fist—before it is stretched out by food. Put less food on your plate than you think you will eat. Use a smaller plate. As soon as you feel full, stop eating and put the timer on for five minutes. When the timer rings, you shouldn't feel hungry anymore since it takes a little while for your brain to recognize your stomach reached its capacity. If you stop eating at the first sign you feel the sensation of fullness, in five minutes your brain receptors catch up with the feeling in your stomach.

Eating Out

Realistically, you won't be able to prepare meals at home all the time. Our lives are busy and many days we are unable to eat at home. Let's first address fast food. Most fast-food restaurants provide a selection of healthy options to choose from, such as a fresh salad with raw ingredients. However, be sure to use either no dressing or as small a portion as you can. If you use more than one fast-food package of salad dressing, you just made your positive eating choice into a negative one. I ask for the salad dressing on the side, and I dip my fork into the dressing before placing food on the fork. That way I get a smaller but flavorful amount of the high-calorie, high-sugar condiment.

Healthy eating choices at a dine-in restaurant are a vegetable plate, fish, or chicken. First, check the menu for the ingredients in your meal choice, and make sure you ask for your food to be served in the healthiest way: no sauces and baked or grilled instead of fried. When your food arrives, the serving size may be substantial. Therefore, when served a large plate of food, before you begin eating, determine how much you will eat to prevent overeating. You might even ask for a to-go container at the beginning of your meal to store what you will not eat at this meal. It is difficult to stop unless you establish boundaries before you begin eating delicious foods.

	Breakfast	Lunch	Snack	Dinner
Food				
Time				
Three Hours Since Last Meal?				
Hungry?				
Feel an Emotion? Describe:				
Satisfied or Stuffed				
Digestive Issue?				
Poor Mental Clarity?				
Bad Mood?				

33

DAY 33: 80/20 PERCENT RULE

Guide your eating with the 80/20 percent rule. *If you eat healthy 80 percent of the time and not so healthy 20 percent of the time, this will probably be an improvement.* I don't eat perfectly, but with God's help I try. If I mess up, the next day I get to start new, as indicated in:

Because of the LORD's great love we are not consumed,
    for his compassions never fail.
    They are new every morning;
    great is your faithfulness.

Lamentations 3:22–23 (NIV)

Each morning as I wake up, my body tells me how well I ate the previous day. If I did not experience any blood sugar fluctuations, I have a clear mind and abundant energy. The incredible sensation of how God created our bodies to feel motivates me to continue to eat well every day. I am more productive when I eat healthy foods.

However, don't make your expectations too high. Remember the 80/20 rule: if you improve your eating 80 percent of the time, you will improve your diet. This lifestyle change is not an all-or-nothing situation. If you don't follow healthy dietary guidelines 100 percent of the time, don't adopt the belief that you failed. Instead, give yourself grace as God does. Try to do well, but if you don't eat correctly 20 percent of the time, that's okay. It's still probably better than the way you were eating before. Get back on track as soon as you can.

	Breakfast	Lunch	Snack	Dinner
Food				
Time				
Three Hours Since Last Meal?				
Hungry?				
Feel an Emotion? Describe:				
Satisfied or Stuffed				
Digestive Issue?				
Poor Mental Clarity?				
Bad Mood?				

34

DAY 34: JOURNAL TIME

	Breakfast	Lunch	Snack	Dinner
Food				
Time				
Three Hours Since Last Meal?				
Hungry?				
Feel an Emotion? Describe:				
Satisfied or Stuffed				
Digestive Issue?				
Poor Mental Clarity?				
Bad Mood?				

35

DAY 35: SABBATH REFLECTIONS

	Breakfast	Lunch	Snack	Dinner
Food				
Time				
Three Hours Since Last Meal?				
Hungry?				
Feel an Emotion? Describe:				
Satisfied or Stuffed				
Digestive Issue?				
Poor Mental Clarity?				
Bad Mood?				

PART VI
WEEK 6

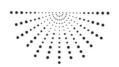

MENU PLAN

WEEKLY MENU PLANNING

When you plan your menu, choose a pleasant spot (outside, by a fire, coffee shop). This may take up to an hour, but is well worth your time and effort. Use the recipes in appendix 4 of *7 Steps to Get Off Sugar and Carbohydrates* (SusanUNeal.com/appendix), another healthy cookbook, or an app on your smartphone to find recipes. I provided a list of healthy food options in appendix 3 to give you ideas of what to cook. Post your menu on the refrigerator, so you know what you planned to cook for each meal during the week.

Cooking from scratch is important. For example, do not buy garlic already minced in a jar. You have no idea how old it is. The nutrients from fruits and vegetables begin to break down as soon as you cut them. Instead, mince a fresh clove of garlic.

It might take longer to cook from scratch, but the food will be more nutritious and low in sugar. Your health is worth it. Your family will appreciate the time you invest into preparing healthy, delicious meals. Make the transition from eating convenience foods, such as processed foods, take out, or eating out, to home cooked food.

Use the following chart to plan out your weekly menu.

Meal	Monday	Tuesday
Breakfast		
Lunch		
Snack		
Dinner		

Meal	Wednesday	Thursday
Breakfast		
Lunch		
Snack		
Dinner		

Meal	Friday	Saturday
Breakfast		
Lunch		
Snack		
Dinner		

Meal	Sunday
Breakfast	
Lunch	
Snack	
Dinner	

WELL-BEING CHART

The following Well-Being Chart will help you determine how habits affect your well-being. Record the number of hours you slept and add a Y for yes and N for no for the other items tracked below. Recognize if there is a correlation between your energy level and mood with the consumption of unhealthy foods. List those foods on the chart.

Your sleep and diet affect your brain. If you slept less than eight hours or ate unhealthy foods, color the box red in the Well-Being Chart. If you experience a day with high energy and clarity of mind color the corresponding boxes green.

Many of the symptoms listed in the Well-Being Chart (energy, brain fog, mood, anxiety, irritability, digestive issues) are affected by the foods you consume.

At the end of the week review your Daily Food Journals and compare it with your Well-Being Chart to determine how you did food wise along with the corresponding symptoms. When you color boxes red (negative symptoms) and green (positive symptoms) it is easier to figure out what type of food makes your body function well and vice-versa. When you find a food culprit, eliminate it from your diet.

Please complete the information below.

Days	36	37	38	39	40	41	42
Hours of Sleep							
Ate Unhealthy Foods: List the foods							
Binged							
Low Energy Level							
Brain Fog							
Bad Mood							
Anxiety							
Irritable							
Digestive Issues							
Physical Activity							
Probiotics							
Spent Time w/ God							

36

DAY 36: EXERCISE

It doesn't matter what type of exercise you do as long as you do it. Walking, lifting weights, or taking a group fitness class are a few examples of healthy exercise. After you improve your eating habits and begin feeling better, try to exercise for twenty minutes three times a week. Even if you only walk down the road a couple of blocks and come back, start moving.

Record the exercise you perform in the Fitness Tracker chart in this journal. If you haven't been exercising, determine why. Is it because you don't have the time? Or are you too tired?

Is there a type of physical endeavor you enjoyed when you were younger? Maybe it's time to try it again. I enjoyed swimming as a child, so I try to swim laps in my pool a couple of times a week. Figure out what you like to do and put it on your calendar. Ask a family member, friend, neighbor, or even your accountability partner to join you on a regular basis, so you can encourage each other to keep up this beneficial habit.

Exercise is a positive coping strategy for dealing with stress; it burns off adrenaline and improves sleep. Do you engage in relaxation techniques such as Christian yoga or meditation? Yoga eases pain, improves depression, and boosts metabolism and immunity. Yoga and meditation calm the mind and body. I created several Christian yoga products including DVDs, books, and card decks available at Christianyoga.com.

Do you routinely exercise? If yes, what type of activity do you perform? Do you enjoy this type of exercise?

_____

If you do not routinely exercise, what type of workout do you enjoy?

_____

How can you incorporate an enjoyable form of activity into your life?

_____

_____

	Breakfast	Lunch	Snack	Dinner
Food				
Time				
Three Hours Since Last Meal?				
Hungry?				
Feel an Emotion? Describe:				
Satisfied or Stuffed				
Digestive Issue?				
Poor Mental Clarity?				
Bad Mood?				

37

DAY 37: PRACTICE GRATITUDE

When you embrace a mind-set of gratitude, dopamine releases in your brain. Remember that dopamine, the feel-good neurohormone, releases when you eat sugar and wheat. Instead of getting the positive feeling from a bad habit, get it from a good one—by journaling gratefulness. Next time you want to eat something unhealthy, grab this journal instead and record what you are grateful for in the Gratitude Log at the beginning of this book.

To get an into an attitude of gratitude, I listen to praise music, whether I am cooking, driving, or getting ready for work. Listening to worship music gets me into the mood to praise God. That's when dopamine releases and I feel the Holy Spirit's vibrancy within me. Fill your mind, heart, and body with the Spirit of God by putting the right things in your spirit.

Fix your thoughts on what is true and good and right. Think about things that are pure and lovely, and dwell on the fine, good things in others. Think about all you can praise God for and be glad about.

Philippians 4:8 (TLB)

Lord,

I want to focus my thoughts on "what is true and good and right," not on negative things. Help me to change my mind-set and priorities so I focus on the things that are important to you. Thank you for giving me gladness when I praise you! Jesus, through your name I pray. Amen.

Journal about what you are grateful for:

_____

_____

_____

_____

_____

_____

	Breakfast	Lunch	Snack	Dinner
Food				
Time				
Three Hours Since Last Meal?				
Hungry?				
Feel an Emotion? Describe:				
Satisfied or Stuffed				
Digestive Issue?				
Poor Mental Clarity?				
Bad Mood?				

DAY 38: FRUIT OF THE SPIRIT: SELF-CONTROL

Another reason some people struggle to eat healthy foods is their bodies betray their mental commitment. It may not be just a matter of self-control; you may have a food addiction (day 9) or overgrowth of Candida (day 10) in the GI tract that causes you to overeat. There could also be an emotional connection to food (day 22). Finding out the root issue is instrumental to being freed from the compulsion to overeat.

We need to recognize how addictions affect us physically, so we can be prepared with the mental ammunition needed to stay strong. Food addiction is quite prevalent in our society today. It is a biochemical disorder that cannot be controlled through self-control. An addiction causes a person to repeat the same type of behavior despite life-damaging consequences. That is why we need to learn to use God's spiritual weapons.

Have you ever relied on self-control to overcome temptations of the flesh but failed? We need to use God's power to conquer temptations and food issues. How do we access his power? Let's look for the answer in the Bible. Speak these verses out loud:

. . .

In your hands are strength and power
    to exalt and give strength to all.

1 Chronicles 29:12 (NIV)

You are their glorious strength.
    It pleases you to make us strong.

Psalm 89:17

From these verses, we see that "the Lord" can "give strength to all" and it pleases him "to make us strong." The transformation from food addiction cannot come from dietary boundaries and self-control alone; it must come from God helping you. Turn to the Lord when you want to eat inappropriately. Explore your emotions with him and ask him to stabilize your feelings. Allow him to minister to your heart and mind, and your eating habits will improve.

Have you tried to overcome inappropriate eating before? If you failed, you were probably dealing with the issue through your own resolve. Instead, call on the power of the Holy Spirit to change you from the inside out. With God's help, you can overcome and succeed.

The Lord hears his people when they call to him for help.
    He rescues them from all their troubles.
    The Lord is close to the brokenhearted;
    he rescues those whose spirits are crushed.
    The righteous person faces many troubles,
    but the Lord comes to the rescue each time.

Psalm 34:17–19

Ask God to help you overcome your struggle with food.

_____

_____

_____

Psalm 89:17 states that it pleases God to make us strong. So ask him to give you his supernatural strength to make healthy eating choices and not fall prey to temptations.

_____

_____

_____

Lord,

I know you hear me when I call for help, so I am asking you to rescue me from my struggles with food. Strengthen me each time I am tempted. Please help me to remember to always call upon you. Thank you. In Jesus's name, I pray. Amen.

	Breakfast	Lunch	Snack	Dinner
Food				
Time				
Three Hours Since Last Meal?				
Hungry?				
Feel an Emotion? Describe:				
Satisfied or Stuffed				
Digestive Issue?				
Poor Mental Clarity?				
Bad Mood?				

DAY 39: PLAN FOR THE PITFALLS

No one is perfect. You will have days when you eat sugar, wheat, or processed foods. That's okay. This happens to everyone; don't let it discourage you. Share your feelings with your accountability/prayer partner. Pray together. Please join my closed Facebook group, 7 Steps to Get Off Sugar, Carbs, and Gluten and share with me how you are doing. If you would like healthy living tips please like my Facebook page at Facebook.com/HealthyLivingSeries/.

Changing the way you eat will be a challenging task, but one you can conquer. If you relapse, get up, brush the dust off yourself, and start again. Realize what triggered your cravings. Was it your emotions? Did you write about your feelings, obstacles, and victories in the sixth and seventh days of this journal? These pages were left blank for that purpose.

Did you complete your Daily Food Journal and record when you overate in the Binge Eating Tracker? Have you figured out what triggered you to overeat, and what you might do the next time you are tempted by recording it in the Temptation/Struggle Log? Through journaling you can identify your triggers and strategize how to avoid them. By now you should be well on your way to figuring out your health puzzle.

It is normal for people to stay the course and then fall off the wagon and binge. This cycle continues to repeat itself, but as you continue to turn to God and rely on his strength, slowly but surely you will gain control of your body, mind, and spirit. The changes in your eating habits are a lifelong lifestyle journey so you can live the abundant life Jesus wants you to experience. Not a life filled with disease and unwanted, unhealthy symptoms.

If you did not track everything in this journal but still want to make further improvements in your health and weight, go back and fill in the charts. If you do you will get positive results.

Make check marks by the charts you completed in this journal:

Gratitude Log

Victory Log

Temptation/Struggle Log

Binge Eating Tracker

Issue Tracker

New Healthy Living Habits Log

Water Tracker

Steps Tracker

Fitness Tracker

Well-Being Chart

Daily Food Journal

Appendix 2: My Battle Strategies Plan

I am proud of you for your effort. May God bless your endeavor to improve your health and well-being.

	Breakfast	Lunch	Snack	Dinner
Food				
Time				
Three Hours Since Last Meal?				
Hungry?				
Feel an Emotion? Describe:				
Satisfied or Stuffed				
Digestive Issue?				
Poor Mental Clarity?				
Bad Mood?				

DAY 40: IMPROVE YOUR HEALTH

After six weeks I hope you feel like a new person. Hopefully some bothersome symptoms have already disappeared, as well as some excess weight. Maybe big chores, like house cleaning, don't seem so difficult anymore, or perhaps you feel like putting on a cute outfit and attending a social event. As you continue to nourish your body, weak-functioning cells will be replaced by new ones, and your body will work to heal itself of diseases the way the Lord intended.

As a certified health and wellness coach, I encourage and guide others to regain their health. A client told me her pediatric endocrinologist diagnosed her son as obese and prediabetic. We reviewed the types of food her family ate and developed a plan to cut out unhealthy foods. She resolved to eliminate wheat, milk, and fruit juice from her family's diet. I encouraged her to try to improve their eating habits 80 percent of the time and not worry about what they ate the other 20 percent of the time, since no one can be perfect. If you would like me to assist you on this journey to improve your health as your wellness coach go to SusanUNeal.com/Health-Coaching. May God bless your endeavor to improve your health.

. . .

Dear friend, I hope all is well with you and that you are as healthy in body as you are strong in spirit.

3 John 2

Lord,

It is my greatest desire that this journal strengthened my fellow brothers and sisters in Christ. Please help the reader to put the health puzzle together so he or she may experience the abundant life you designed. Bless all those who read this journal.

Thank you. In Jesus's name, I pray. Amen.

	Breakfast	Lunch	Snack	Dinner
Food				
Time				
Three Hours Since Last Meal?				
Hungry?				
Feel an Emotion? Describe:				
Satisfied or Stuffed				
Digestive Issue?				
Poor Mental Clarity?				
Bad Mood?				

41

DAY 41: JOURNAL TIME

	Breakfast	Lunch	Snack	Dinner
Food				
Time				
Three Hours Since Last Meal?				
Hungry?				
Feel an Emotion? Describe:				
Satisfied or Stuffed				
Digestive Issue?				
Poor Mental Clarity?				
Bad Mood?				

42

DAY 42: SABBATH REFLECTIONS

	Breakfast	Lunch	Snack	Dinner
Food				
Time				
Three Hours Since Last Meal?				
Hungry?				
Feel an Emotion? Describe:				
Satisfied or Stuffed				
Digestive Issue?				
Poor Mental Clarity?				
Bad Mood?				

APPENDIX 1: FOOD ADDICTION BATTLE STRATEGIES

1. Complete the logs, charts, and journaling sections of this book.
2. Ask a friend to be your accountability and prayer partner.
3. Find a specific Bible verse to oppose your food issue, write it on an index card, and memorize it. Speak the verse out loud every time you feel the urge to eat unhealthy foods.
4. Determine food triggers by writing them down in the Temptation/Struggle Log and avoid the trigger.
5. Record every time you overeat in the Binge Eating Tracker.
6. When you are tempted to overeat or eat unhealthy food:

- pray
- go for a walk
- recite your Bible verse
- call your prayer partner
- drink two glasses of water
- listen to praise music and worship God
- spend time with and meditate about God
- write in this journal

7. When you eat any unhealthy food, be sure to journal afterward—every single time. Figure out what you told yourself that validated why it was okay to eat the item. Then go through the Five Spiritual Steps to Freedom from Addiction. If you journal and implement this five-step plan every time you binge, you will experience success. This is part of retraining your mind.

8. Implement the Five Spiritual Steps to Freedom from Addiction:

- Name what controls you.
- Submit yourself completely to God.
- Use the name of Jesus.
- Use the Word of God.
- Praise God and practice gratitude.

Complete the study *Christian Study Guide for 7 Steps to Get Off Sugar and Carbohydrates.*

APPENDIX 2: MY BATTLE STRATEGIES PLAN

1.

2.

3.

4.

5.

6.

7.

8.

9.

10.

APPENDIX 3: HEALTHY FOOD OPTIONS

The following daily meal categories include a list of appropriate healthy food options for your menu planning and shopping lists.

Breakfast

- oatmeal with pecans and cinnamon
- pancakes made with almond flour (recipe link: Pinterest.com/SusanUNeal/breakfast/)
- quinoa with a smashed banana, almond milk, and walnuts
- scrambled eggs with hash browns
- omelet with green onions, red peppers, and mushrooms
- berries with plain Greek yogurt
- chia parfait with fruit
- homemade granola with berries and/or Greek yogurt
- hash browns with onions, peppers, and a sliced avocado on top
- mashed avocado with two fried eggs on top
- pancakes made with two eggs and one smashed banana

Lunch

- a salad or vegetable plate, if eating out
- romaine lettuce wrap sandwich with any meat or vegetable
- cucumber sandwich—cut a cucumber in half and load it with meat (not processed packaged lunch meat) and veggies
- salad with fish, chicken, nuts, or avocado
- baked potato bar with olive oil, broccoli, scallions, and sunflower seeds
- guacamole or hummus with sliced vegetables
- whole avocado and an heirloom tomato
- baked sweet potato with butter, cinnamon, and honey

Snack

- sliced green apple with almond or cashew butter
- berries with whipped cream made with coconut milk
- raw vegetables with hummus or guacamole
- boiled egg or deviled eggs (made with organic mayonnaise)
- carrots and celery sticks
- berries with slivered almonds
- nuts—raw almonds, pecans, pistachios, macadamia nuts, or cashews
- organic popcorn popped on the stove (not microwave popcorn)

Dinner

- chicken fajitas with guacamole, lettuce, tomato, and avocado on a coconut tortilla wrap (available at health food stores)
- spaghetti with a baked spaghetti squash for the noodles
- steak, mushrooms, green beans with slivered almonds, and a salad
- salmon, sautéed red cabbage, and wild rice
- baked or grilled chicken, quinoa, and sautéed or grilled zucchini and yellow squash

- chili made with lean meat
- fish, salad, and asparagus
- beef stew with potato, carrots, celery, bok choy, and onions
- black bean soup
- fresh field peas with sliced tomatoes, fried okra, and corn pone bread (recipe in appendix 4 of *7 Steps to Get Off Sugar and Carbohydrates*. You can obtain a printable version of this appendix at SusanUNeal.com/appendix).
- shrimp fettuccine alfredo with shirataki noodles, and a salad
- roasted whole chicken with onions, potatoes, carrots, and bok choy
- salad with berries, nuts, and seeds

Dessert

- dark chocolate (at least 70 percent chocolate)
- dark chocolate almond cookies (recipe in appendix 4 of *7 Steps to Get Off Sugar and Carbohydrates*)
- chocolate nut clusters
- dark chocolate–covered strawberries
- one dried date to seven pecan halves (be careful, as dates are high in sugar)

NOTES

Well-Being Chart
1. Dale E. Bredesen, Edwin C. Amos, Jonathan Canick, Mary Ackerley, Cyrus Raji, Milan Fiala, and Jamila Ahdidan, "Reversal of cognitive decline in Alzheimer's disease," *Aging*, June 2016.

Daily Food Journal
2. Ibid.

Day 3: Healthy Eating Guidelines
3. John Brennan, "What is Roundup Ready Corn," Sciencing, April 25, 2017

Day 10: Candida
4. "Candida Yeast Infection, Leaky Gut, Irritable Bowel and Food Allergies," National Candida Center, https://www.nationalcandida-center.com/Leaky-Gut-and-Candida-Yeast-Infection-s/1823.htm.

Day 12: Foods to Eliminate
5. Stacy Simon, "World Health Organization Says Processed Meat Causes Cancer," *American Cancer Society*, October 26, 2015,

https://www.cancer.org/latest-news/world-health-organization-says-processed-meat-causes-cancer.html.

Day 19: Five Spiritual Steps to Freedom from Addiction
  6. Larry Lea, *The Weapons of Your Warfare: Equipping Yourself to Defeat the Enemy* (Reading: Cox and Wyman, Ltd. 1990), 126, 182.

ABOUT THE AUTHOR

Susan U. Neal, RN, MBA, MHS, is an award-winning author, speaker, and certified health and wellness coach whose background in nursing and health services led her to seek new ways to educate and coach people to overcome health challenges. She published the award-winning book *7 Steps to Get Off Sugar and Carbohydrates* and its corresponding Bible study *Christian Study Guide for 7 Steps to Get Off Sugar and Carbohydrates*. Her other books include, *Solving the Gluten Puzzle*, *Scripture Yoga*, a #1 Amazon best-seller, and *Yoga for Beginners*. Her passion and mission is to help others improve their health and weight. To learn more about Susan visit her website at SusanUNeal.com.

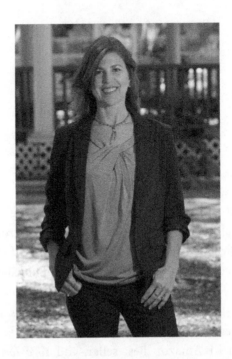

Susan has been interviewed on the *Bridges Show* on Christian Television Network (CTN), Moody Radio, Blog Talk Radio, and Premier Christian Radio from the UK.

Susan founded Scripture Yoga™, a form of Christian yoga, and enjoys leading classes at her church and fitness club. She is a speaker and enjoys teaching Scripture Yoga™ sessions at women's retreats, Christian conferences, and yoga retreats.

Previously Susan worked as a kidney transplant nurse at Shands Hospital in Gainesville, Florida; assistant administrator at Mayo Clinic Jacksonville; and quality assurance nurse at Blue Cross Blue Shield of Florida. Currently, she owns her own business, Christian Yoga, LLC, and publishes Christian products, along with teaching group fitness classes.

Connect with Susan Online

Susan created the Healthy Living Series blog to provide healthy lifestyle tips and the latest scientific findings regarding foods and health. She also posts menu and grocery shopping list to help with planning healthy menus. You can subscribe to the blog at Susan-UNeal.com/healthy-living-blog.

You can follow Susan on:
    Facebook.com/SusanUllrichNeal
    Facebook.com/ScriptureYoga/
    Facebook.com/HealthyLivingSeries/
    Twitter.com/SusanNealYoga
    Youtube.com/c/SusanNealScriptureYoga/
    Pinterest.com/SusanUNeal/
    Instagram.com/healthylivingseries/
    Linkedin.com/in/susannealyoga/

Follow Susan on BookBub to get an email when she releases a new book or her books go on sale at BookBub.com/authors/susan-u-neal.

SusanUNeal.com and ChristianYoga.com
SusanNeal@bellsouth.net

OTHER PRODUCTS BY SUSAN NEAL

HEALTHY LIVING SERIES COURSE & BOOKS

7 Steps to Reclaim Your Health and Optimal Weight Online Course

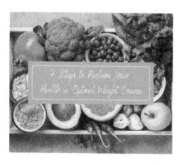

If you need additional support making this lifestyle change, purchase my course, 7 Steps to Reclaim Your Health and Optimal Weight at Susan-UNeal.com/courses/7-steps-to-get-off-sugar-and-carbs-course. In this course I walk you through all the material covered in my Healthy Living Series.

I teach you the root causes of inappropriate eating habits and help you resolve those issues. One solved, taming your appetite is much easier. Learn how to change your eating habits successfully once and for all.

Book 1: *7 Steps to Get Off Sugar and Carbohydrates*

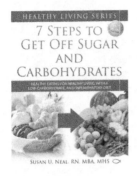

SUSAN U. NEAL, RN, MBA, MHS

Over half of Americans live with a chronic illness and forty percent suffer from obesity, primarily due to the overconsumption of sugar and refined carbohydrates. *Seven Steps to Get Off Sugar and Carbohydrates* provides a day-by-day plan to wean your body off these addictive products and regain your health. These changes in your eating habits will start your lifestyle journey to the abundant life Jesus wants you to experience, not a life filled with disease and poor health.

You will learn how to:

- eliminate brain fog, cure diseases, and lose weight
- choose foods that benefit versus foods that damage—the ones God gave us to eat, not the food industry
- find healthy food alternatives and plan your menu
- recognize the emotional reasons we overeat and the science behind food addiction and a candida infection (overgrowth of yeast in the gut)
- identify food triggers and use God's Word to fight impulsive eating
- locate resources—educational videos and books, meal planning, support organizations, and recipes.

Jesus said in John 10:10, "The thief's purpose is to steal, kill and destroy. My purpose is to give life in all its fullness" (TLB). Are you living life in its fullness? Is your health or weight impeding you from embracing a healthy, bountiful life? If you take these simple seven steps, you will regain the life God created you for. You will love the new you! To purchase go to ChristianYoga.com/yoga-books-decks.

Christian Study Guide for 7 Steps to Get Off Sugar and Carbohydrates

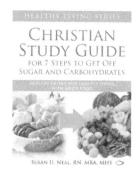

More than half of Americans suffer with a chronic disease and 40 percent are obese. Struggling with health problems is not our true destiny. Jesus promised us a life of abundance. He also told us, "The thief's purpose is to steal, kill, and destroy" (John 10:10 TLB). Shortening our lifespan through our unhealthy food patterns is the enemy's perfect scheme.

Many of the health problems we suffer are connected to eating habits. Change your life by changing the types of food you eat. Learn which foods are beneficial and which foods make you sick. Don't struggle on your own to make necessary lifestyle changes. Learn how to mobilize God's power. Through the Holy Spirit, you become strong and able to accomplish what you cannot achieve by your own efforts. When you apply God's wisdom, along with accurate knowledge about today's food, you will improve your health and weight and defeat the enemy.

This study guide provides a group experience to help implement the plans in *7 Steps to Get Off Sugar and Carbohydrates*. Accountability and encouragement improve your chance for success as you learn to become a healthy steward of the resources you've been given. You only have one body, and you want it to carry you through this life gracefully. Reclaim the abundant life God wants you to live. Take this journey to recover your health and achieve all the blessings the Lord has in store for you.

Healthy Living Series: 3 Books in 1: 7 Steps to Get Off Sugar and Carbohydrates; Christian Study Guide for 7 Steps to Get Off Sugar and Carbohydrates; Healthy Living Journal

This mega book contains all three of the Healthy Living Series books:

7 Steps to Get Off Sugar and Carbohydrates
Christian Study Guide for 7 Steps to Get Off Sugar and Carbohydrates
Healthy Living Journal.

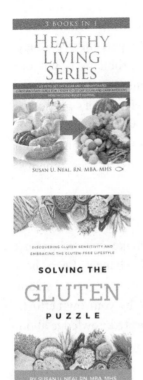

Solving the Gluten Puzzle

Are you experiencing symptoms that you or your doctor don't understand? Ruling out a gluten-related diagnosis may move you one step closer to wellness. Discovering whether you have celiac disease, gluten sensitivity, wheat sensitivity, or a wheat allergy is like piecing together a puzzle. Random pieces don't make sense and won't until the whole picture fits together. *Solving the Gluten Puzzle* explains the symptoms, diagnostic tests, and treatment for these ailments.

Nearly 10 percent of the population is affected by one of four gluten-related disorders, which can cause more than two hundred symptoms, most of which are not digestive. These disorders can strike at any age. Unfortunately, a single diagnostic test to determine gluten sensitivity does not exist. Consequently, up to 80 percent of individuals go undiagnosed. Determine whether you suffer from one of these conditions and how to cure your symptoms by embracing a gluten-free lifestyle.

HOW TO PREVENT, IMPROVE, AND REVERSE ALZHEIMER'S AND DEMENTIA

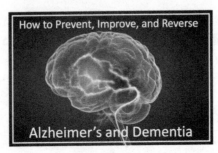

This pamphlet provides twenty-four interventions you can do to prevent, improve, or even reverse Alzheimer's and dementia. There is finally hope. To order this pamphlet go to SusanUNeal.com/appendix.

YOGA BOOKS

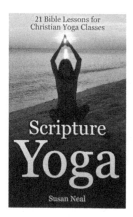

Scripture Yoga assists yoga students in creating a Christian atmosphere for their classes. Choose from twenty-one lessons, each a mini–Bible study that will deepen the participants' walk with God.

Each lesson contains a scriptural theme designed to facilitate meditation on God's Word. The Scripture verses are arranged progressively to facilitate an understanding of each Bible study topic. The Bible lessons will enhance the spiritual depth of your yoga class and make it appropriate and desirable for Christian participants.

Check your poses with photographs of over sixty yoga postures taken on the sugar-white sands of the Emerald Coast of Florida. A detailed description of each pose is provided with full-page photographs so postures are easily seen and replicated. You can purchase these books at ChristianYoga.com/yoga-books-decks.

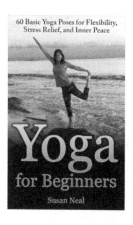

Yoga for Beginners eases you into the inner peace you long for at an easy, step-by-step beginner's pace. Through Susan's gentle encouragement, you will learn how to improve your flexibility and relieve stress. A broad range of yoga poses provides many options for the beginner- to intermediate-level student.

In *Yoga for Beginners* you get it more than basic yoga postures. You will begin to breathe a new sense of well-being when you follow Susan's life-changing eating practices. Learn not only what to eat but also why. This book includes:

1. Sixty basic yoga poses with full-page photographs and detailed explanations
2. Three different routines to give variety
3. Warm-up stretches
4. Injury prevention and posture modification suggestions
5. How to ease pain and anxiety
6. Essential components of yoga such as breathing and stretching
7. Meditation techniques to reduce stress
8. Low-glycemic diet guidelines to obtain optimal weight
9. Causes of sugar cravings and solutions for controlling them

CHRISTIAN YOGA CARD DECKS

Scripture Yoga Card Decks include a yoga pose on one side and a theme-based Bible verse on the other. The decks assist Christian yoga instructors and students in creating a Christian atmosphere for their classes through meditating on the Word of God. You can order the card decks at ChristianYoga.com/yoga-books-decks.

The Fruit of the Spirit Deck

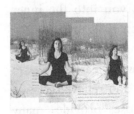
This lesson, The Fruit of the Spirit, describes each of the fruits of the spirit including love, joy, peace, patience, kindness, goodness, gentleness, faithfulness, and self-control. It is a mini– Bible study that will deepen the participants' walk with God.

The Scripture verses are arranged progressively to facilitate a complete understanding of the Bible study topic. The Bible lesson will enhance the spiritual depth of your yoga class, and make it appropriate and desirable for Christian participants.

How to Receive God's Peace Deck

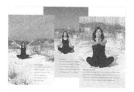

This lesson, How to Receive God's Peace, walks the participant through the steps needed to cast fear and anxiety on God and receive his peace. It is a peace the world cannot give. This mini–Bible study will deepen the participants' walk with God.

SCRIPTURE YOGA DVDS

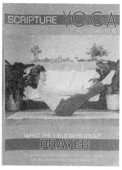

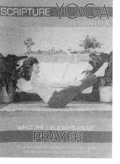

What The Bible Says about Prayer

In this session we explore different aspects of prayer. We look at the "when, where, and how" of prayer illustrated through Bible verses and stories. In this DVD, I share with you many facets of prayer. Prayer is more powerful than we can imagine. This DVD will help your prayer life. To purchase go to Christianyoga.com/dvd-products.

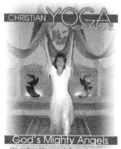

God's Mighty Angels Christian Yoga DVD

Enter the realm of God's mighty angels and find out how they intercede in our lives. Angels are God's messengers and he sends them to protect you wherever you go (Psalm 91:11). Over twenty verses about angels are recited during the class. This is a gentle yoga class that includes twenty-five minutes of stretching and fifty-five minutes of yoga postures for an eighty-minute class. To purchase go to ChristianYoga.com/dvd-products.

Made in the USA
Monee, IL
28 July 2024

62836373R00351